Find surgical videos for *Cholesteatoma* online at MediaCenter.thieme.com!

Simply visit **MediaCenter.thieme.com** and, when prompted during the registration process, enter the scratch-off code below to get started today.

This book cannot be returned once this panel has been scratched off.

In these unique videos the authors discuss real-world cases and demonstrate surgical techniques. The videos illustrate the management of specific clinical scenarios, including disease complications, and clarify surgical procedures. The authors perform surgery on challenging cases, describing how they would handle removal of residual cholesteatoma from a bare faical nerve, how they handle an intact ossicular chain, and much more.

System requirements:

	WINDOWS	MAC	TABLET
Recommended Browser(s)**	Microsoft Internet Explorer 8.0 or later, Firefox 3.x	Firefox 3.x, Safari 4.x	HTML5 mobile browser. iPad — Safari. Opera Mobile — Tablet PCs preferred.
	** all browsers should have JavaScript enabled		
Flash Player Plug-in	Flash Player 9 or Higher* ** Mac users: ATI Rage 128 GPU does not support full-screen mode with hardware scaling*		Tablet PCs with Android OS support Flash 10.1
Minimum Hardware Configurations	Intel® Pentium® II 450 MHz, AMD Athlon™ 600 MHz or faster processor (or equivalent) 512 MB of RAM	PowerPC® G3 500 MHz or faster processor Intel Core™ Duo 1.33 GHz or faster processor 512MB of RAM	Minimum CPU powered at 800MHz 256MB DDR2 of RAM
Recommended for optimal usage experience	Monitor resolutions: • Normal (4:3) 1024×768 or Higher • Widescreen (16:9) 1280×720 or Higher • Widescreen (16:10) 1440×900 or Higher DSL/Cable internet connection at a minimum speed of 384.0 Kbps or faster WiFi 802.11 b/g preferred.		7-inch and 10-inch tablets on maximum resolution. WiFi connection is required.

Cholesteatoma

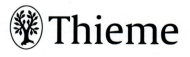

Cholesteatoma

Eric E. Smouha, MD, FACS
Associate Professor
Department of Otolaryngology
Mount Sinai School of Medicine
Director of Otology and Neurotology
Mount Sinai Medical Center
New York, New York

Dennis I. Bojrab, MD
CEO and Director of Research
Michigan Ear Institute
Professor and Chairman of Otolaryngology
Oakland University William Beaumont School of Medicine
Royal Oak, Michigan
Clinical Professor of Otolaryngology and Neurosurgery
Wayne State University School of Medicine
Detroit, Michigan
Neuroscience Co-Director
St. John Providence Health System
Novi, Michigan
Founding President
American CISEPO (Canada International Scientific Exchange Program)
Farmington Hills, Michigan

Thieme
New York • Stuttgart

Thieme Medical Publishers, Inc.
333 Seventh Ave.
New York, NY 10001

Executive Editor: Timothy Hiscock
Managing Editor: J. Owen Zurhellen
Editorial Assistant: Elizabeth D'Ambrosio
Editorial Director: Michael Wachinger
Production Editor: Print Matters, Inc.
International Production Director: Andreas Schabert
Vice President, International Marketing and Sales: Cornelia Schulze
Chief Financial Officer: Sarah Vanderbilt
President: Brian D. Scanlan
Compositor: The Manila Typesetting Co.
Printer: Everbest Printing Company, Ltd.

Library of Congress Cataloging-in-Publication Data
Smouha, Eric E.
Cholesteatoma / Eric E. Smouha, Dennis I. Bojrab.
       p. ; cm.
    Includes bibliographical references and index.
    ISBN 978-1-60406-277-9 (alk. paper)
       1. Cholesteatoma--Surgery. 2. Middle ear--Diseases. I. Bojrab, Dennis I. II. Title.
       [DNLM: 1. Cholesteatoma, Middle Ear--complications. 2. Cholesteatoma, Middle Ear--surgery. WV 230]
    RF229.S46 2010
    617.8'4059--dc22
                                                                                                2010054492

Important note: Medical knowledge is ever-changing. As new research and clinical experience broaden our knowledge, changes in treatment and drug therapy may be required. The authors and editors of the material herein have consulted sources believed to be reliable in their efforts to provide information that is complete and in accord with the standards accepted at the time of publication. However, in view of the possibility of human error by the authors, editors, or publisher of the work herein or changes in medical knowledge, neither the authors, editors, nor publisher, nor any other party who has been involved in the preparation of this work, warrants that the information contained herein is in every respect accurate or complete, and they are not responsible for any errors or omissions or for the results obtained from use of such information. Readers are encouraged to confirm the information contained herein with other sources. For example, readers are advised to check the product information sheet included in the package of each drug they plan to administer to be certain that the information contained in this publication is accurate and that changes have not been made in the recommended dose or in the contraindications for administration. This recommendation is of particular importance in connection with new or infrequently used drugs.

Some of the product names, patents, and registered designs referred to in this book are in fact registered trademarks or proprietary names even though specific reference to this fact is not always made in the text. Therefore, the appearance of a name without designation as proprietary is not to be construed as a representation by the publisher that it is in the public domain.

Printed in China

5 4 3 2 1

ISBN 978-1-60406-277-9

To Lisa,
Thank you for your unwavering support
through this long endeavor.

To Sam and Max,
Always be inquisitive and question everything
until you find *the Way*.

I love you all.

—Eric E. Smouha

To Andria,
I have been Blessed with you in my life. Thank you for sharing my dreams.

To Dennis II, Adrianna, and Andrew,
In life, it's about working hard and sharing your talents.
It's about taking care of your whole self, to then to be able to care for others.
It's about a positive attitude and a heart filled with thankfulness.
May your journey in life be filled with Our Lord's Blessings.

I love all of you very much.

—Dennis I. Bojrab

Contents

Foreword

It is with great pleasure that I endorse this meaningful contribution to the literature in otolaryngology–head and neck surgery. The treatment of cholesteatoma has been an enigma to otolaryngologists for many years. During residency programs, only limited time can be devoted to its medical and surgical management. Eric E. Smouha and Dennis I. Bojrab have organized this unique book to clarify the understanding of cholesteatoma management with one-of-a-kind photos, descriptive artwork, and online surgical videos. They have significantly added to current literature, describing the pathways of spread of cholesteatoma and the surgical and reconstructive approaches used for its management, with particular attention to special situations that one encounters during surgery. Optimal hearing reconstruction is clearly described with photos and online videos.

The brilliant content of this book is based on an instructional course, "Surgical Decision Making in Cholesteatoma," which has been taught (to great interest) at the annual meeting of the American Academy of Otolaryngology–Head and Neck Surgery for more than ten years in order to bring clarity to this complex disease. Each year Dr. Smouha, the moderator of this course, organized relevant case presentations for discussion by experienced otologists with varied backgrounds from different parts of the country. Dr. Bojrab and the other teachers presented their individual approaches to chronic ear problems and debated alternative suggestions, offering the thinking that determined their management choices.

This book and its online content reflect a consensus on some of the basic principles of cholesteatoma management that have been delineated in that course. Drs. Smouha and Bojrab present relevant material commonly faced by otologists and general otolaryngologists in the clinical management of this disease. Organized to be pragmatic and clinically comprehensive, the text provides information and insights useful for achieving better clinical outcomes in the management of patients suffering from cholesteatoma and chronic ear disease. The authors' lengthy experience in the training of residents and fellows has allowed them a wise tutorial approach to the management of the patient with cholesteatoma.

Having myself participated in that AAO-HNS course, I find the different concepts for the management of chronic ear disease presented herein to be very useful in my everyday practice. I fully support the understanding presented in this book; it should be a staple reference for any otolaryngologist–head and neck surgeon.

Simon C. Parisier, MD, FACS
Professor of Otolaryngology, Otology, and Neurotology
New York Eye and Ear Infirmary
New York, New York

Preface

Otolaryngology–head and neck surgery has been a rapidly developing field over the last several years. In fact multiple recognized subspecialties have emerged to cope with the expanded field. Cholesteatoma surgery is still of primary interest for the general otolaryngologist from both a diagnostic and a therapeutic standpoint. We created an instructional course at the American Academy of Otolaryngology–Head and Neck Surgery (AAO-HNS) in 2000, and because of the increasing interest in the care of cholesteatoma seen in our course, it was decided that a comprehensive book on the medical and surgical management of this entity would be appropriate.

Our original concept for the course was to bring together a group of professional colleagues to discuss how they would manage a series of actual cases. We wanted to bring to the audience the challenges of surgical problem solving—using situations actually encountered in the operating room as case examples—while steering clear of dogma. We found it intriguing that the surgeon-panelists, who included Simon Parisier and Barry Hirsch, each with a formidable level of experience and training, would come up with separate approaches to the same clinical problem. Cholesteatoma surgery does not lend itself to a cookbook approach, and there is rarely a situation where one size fits all.

This book is the result of that effort.

Cholesteatoma continues to be a management concern for the general otolaryngologist. This book is organized from a surgical perspective. The first chapter introduces the disease and its general considerations. The next four chapters present the three components of ear surgery, namely, the middle ear, the mastoid, and the meatus and the resultant cavity. Each of these chapters contains a historical overview, a basic review of anatomy and physiology, and a summary of surgical approaches. Chapter 6, Anatomical Issues That Arise at Surgery, is the core of the book. This chapter addresses specific difficulties that arise during surgery, such as labyrinthine fistula and facial nerve dehiscence. The chapter discusses special techniques for handling these situations and provides clini-

cal case examples to demonstrate these principles. Chapter 8, Controversies in Cholesteatoma Surgery, reviews some of the unresolved topics where philosophies of management differ among surgeons, such as the canal wall up versus canal wall down debate, and the value and timing of second-stage surgery. Congenital cholesteatoma is a special topic that is dealt with in Chapter 9. The problem of recidivism is a major one, which frustrates all surgeons who manage cholesteatoma, and this is discussed in Chapter 10. The remainder of the book, Chapters 11 and 12, addresses the complications of otitis media and cholesteatoma surgery.

This book is written for anyone who deals with this unique disease. The scope is meant to be both broad and deep. We hope that this work will become a reference for young surgeons as they become familiar with (and often humbled by) the treatment of this entity, as well as a workbook for experienced practitioners who have to deal with interesting clinical challenges. We hope that we succeed in realizing these objectives here, and we are grateful to our readers for their interest.

◆ Acknowledgments

We are grateful to our wonderful, supportive families who have endured our labor in sharing our experience with you, our readers. We also have gratitude to our respective teachers, as we stand on the shoulders of giants! To Professor Dr. Tauno Palva, for revealing to us the true anatomy of the epitympanum, and for patiently helping us to explain it to others through your assistance with our text and drawings. To Simon Parisier, MD, for providing inspiration and guidance that gave life to this ambitious project and for opening our eyes to new ways of addressing this formidable disease. To Barry Hirsch, MD, for providing original content, criticism, and editorial support, and for always providing an interesting counterpoint to enliven the dialog. To Anthony M. Pazos, whose expertise in medical illustration led to the fantastic artwork that graces these pages.

1

General Considerations in Cholesteatoma

Cholesteatoma is an antiquated term that has persisted through generations of use. Cholesteatoma would have been better named *keratoma*.[1] It is a growth of keratinizing squamous epithelium originating from the external layer of the tympanic membrane or ear canal that invades the middle ear cleft (the air-containing space that is medial to the plane of the tympanic membrane) (**Fig. 1.1**). Cholesteatoma has two components—the acellular keratin *debris*, which forms the contents of the sac, and the *matrix*, which forms the sac itself. The cholesteatoma matrix consists of an inner layer of keratinizing squamous epithelium and an outer layer of subepithelial connective tissue (perimatrix). The matrix is the biologically active component of the cholesteatoma: the epithelial layer produces the keratin, whereas the subepithelial layer contains mesenchymal cells that can resorb bone and that give the cholesteatoma its invasive properties.

Cholesteatoma is a destructive process that invades the middle ear and causes damage by passive growth and active destruction of adjacent bony structures. Cholesteatoma first forms when keratinizing squamous epithelium from the external canal traverses the plane of the tympanic membrane. Once this plane is breached, the cholesteatoma sheds squamous debris into its center and grows passively to occupy the middle ear cleft (which consists of the eustachian tube, middle ear, and mastoid air cell system). But cholesteatoma is not merely a passive process; it is actively invasive. The cholesteatoma matrix produces proteolytic (collagenolytic) enzymes that can erode bone. Cholesteatoma can also become secondarily infected, leading to malodorous discharge.

Cholesteatomas can be congenital or acquired, the latter occurring far more frequently. Acquired cholesteatomas can arise by three pathogenetic mechanisms.[2,3] By far the most common is *retraction*, by which the keratinizing squamous epithelium of the tympanic membrane invaginates into the middle ear from the pars tensa or into the attic (epitympanum) from the pars flaccida (**Fig. 1.2A,B**). Basal hyperplasia may also occur, whereby keratinocytes invade the subepithelium by breaking through the basement membrane.[4] A retraction pocket cholesteatoma is termed a primary ac-

quired cholesteatoma. A second mechanism is by *epithelial migration* from the edges of a tympanic membrane perforation, termed secondary acquired cholesteatoma (**Fig. 1.3**). The third (potential) mechanism is by *squamous metaplasia*, transformation of the nonkeratinizing mucosal lining of the middle ear into keratinizing squamous epithelium (the least common mechanism, and some even doubt that this ever occurs). Congenital cholesteatomas are epithelial rests that become entrapped in the middle ear cleft during embryogenesis.[5] They appear as a keratin sac behind an intact tympanic membrane (**Fig. 1.4**). They are believed to occur from failure of the normal involution of embryonic epidermoid tissue; this squamous epithelium trapped within the middle ear during embryogenesis is most commonly attached to the anterior border of the tensor tympani muscle but may also be attached to the stapedial tendon.

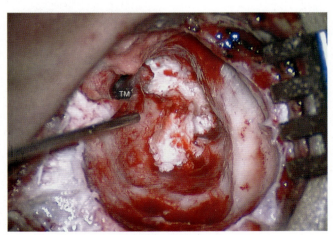

Fig. 1.1 Cholesteatoma should properly be named *keratoma*. It is an epithelial sac containing keratin debris that grows from the eardrum into the mastoid. As shown here, cholesteatoma can attain quite a large size. TM, tympanic membrane.

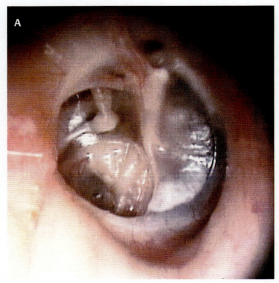
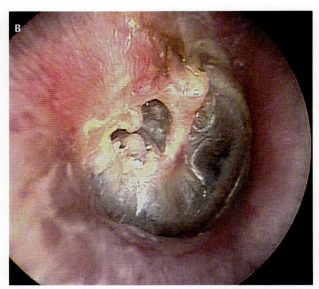

Fig. 1.2 (**A**) Cholesteatoma most commonly arises from a retraction pocket of the pars flaccida or the pars tensa, as shown here. (**B**) Over time, the retraction pocket can become infected, invade the middle ear cleft, erode bone, and liberate keratin. A retraction pocket cholesteatoma is termed primary acquired.

The clinical behavior of cholesteatoma can vary over time. Cholesteatoma may grow insidiously at first, and can attain a significant size without causing any symptoms other than hearing loss (**Fig. 1.5**). Over time, the cholesteatoma will usually become infected, leading to malodorous discharge (**Fig. 1.6**). The discharge may respond to treatment with antibiotic ear drops, but the improvement is usually only temporary. Recurrent or persistent ear discharge should make one suspect cholesteatoma, even when the lesion is not clinically evident.

Bone erosion is responsible for the invasive nature of cholesteatoma.[6-9] Erosion of the lateral epitympanic wall (*scutum*) occurs early as the cholesteatoma expands into the attic (**Fig. 1.7A**). Erosion of the ossicles (the lenticular process of the incus and the superstructure of the stapes) occurs as the cholesteatoma grows into the middle ear, and causes conductive hearing loss (**Fig. 1.7B**). Erosion of the bony septations of the mastoid appears as *coalescence* on computed tomographic (CT) radiographs; this finding, plus scutum erosion, is the radiologic hallmark of cholesteatoma. Erosion

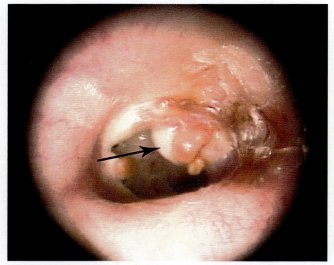

Fig. 1.3   Cholesteatoma may also arise from migration of keratinizing squamous epithelium into the middle ear space from a tympanic membrane perforation (*arrow*). This is termed *secondary acquired* cholesteatoma.

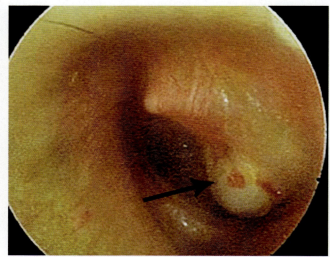

Fig. 1.4   *Congenital* cholesteatoma is an epithelial sac or pearl behind an intact tympanic membrane (*arrow*).

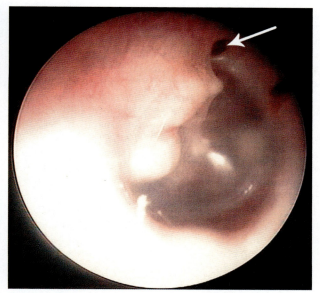

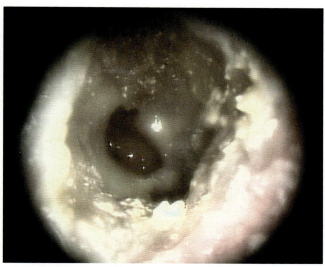

Fig. 1.6 Over time, cholesteatomas usually become infected, leading to malodorous discharge.

Fig. 1.5 Cholesteatoma can grow insidiously. Here a large sac is seen in the middle ear, which arose from a small attic retraction (*arrow*). The patient was a young child who had no hearing loss and no history of infection.

of bony partitions between the mastoid air cell system and inner ear and intracranial structures permit complications to occur (*complications* are defined as spread of disease outside of the pneumatized portions of the temporal bone and include suppurative (coalescent) mastoiditis, labyrinthitis, facial nerve paralysis, petrositis, and intracranial infections).

The treatment of cholesteatoma is surgical, and, although surgery is mandatory, it is not always definitive. The capacity for *recurrence* is another important feature of cholesteatoma that reflects its invasive nature. Recurrence is the regrowth of disease after adequate surgical extirpation. The significant rate of recurrence makes the management of cholesteatoma daunting for the surgeon and frustrating for the patient. Indeed, in the best hands, recurrence rates of up to 30% in adults and up to 70% in children have been reported.

The anatomical patterns of growth of cholesteatoma are determined by the mucosal partitions of the middle ear and attic. A one-cell-thick layer of low cuboidal epithelium lines the middle ear promontory and attic and envelops the

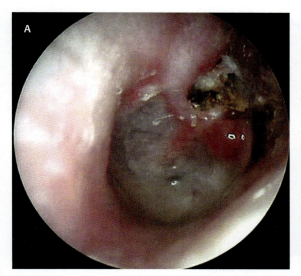

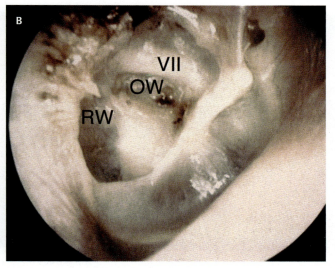

Fig. 1.7 Bone erosion and invasion are the biological hallmarks of cholesteatoma. **(A)** A cholesteatoma that has eroded the scutum (lateral epitympanic bone) to invade the attic. **(B)** A middle ear cholesteatoma that has eaten away the incus and stapes and draped itself onto the facial nerve (VII) and oval (OW) and round windows (RW).

ossicles in the same way that the mesentery envelops the intestines. The mucosal folds form the epitympanic spaces of von Troeltsch, which divide the attic into three spaces: a *lateral epitympanic space* (the Prussak space) situated between the scutum and the malleus head and incus body, the *anterior epitympanic space* demarcated posteriorly by the bony "cog," and the *posterior epitympanic space* surrounding the incus and malleus and leading posteriorly to the aditus ad antrum (**Fig. 1.8A–D**).

The posterior and anterior epitympanic pouches were first described by von Troeltsch,[10] based on the work of Hammar,[11] who in fetuses had described the formation of various epitympanic mucosal folds. Prussak[12] later described the "superior pouch of the tympanic membrane," a small air space that is bounded laterally by the Shrapnell membrane, medially by the malleus neck and head, anteriorly by a membrane toward the anterior pouch, superiorly by the lateral malleal ligamental fold. Posteriorly it is open to the posterior pouch.

(These spaces are illustrated in **Fig. 1.9**.) The Prussak space is thus aerated from the superior portion of the tympanic cavity. Siebenmann[13] in the 19th century summarized the knowledge of the epitympanic folds, pointing attention to a "transverse membrane," the tensor fold, which separates the anterior epitympanum from the supratubal recess. In his drawings he depicted the anterior and posterior pouches and showed the division of the lateral attic into an upper and lower compartment by the thin incudomalleal fold. Aeration of the large epitympanic compartments above the diaphragm, as well as of the antrum and mastoid cells is provided by the tympanic isthmus. The isthmus extends from the posterior medial incudal ligament anteriorly up to the tensor tendon (**Fig. 1.9**).

In 1964, Proctor[14] depicted the anterior, posterior, and lateral epitympanic spaces as he understood them, and for years these illustrations have been widely accepted and used to explain the paths of spread of cholesteatoma. Palva and

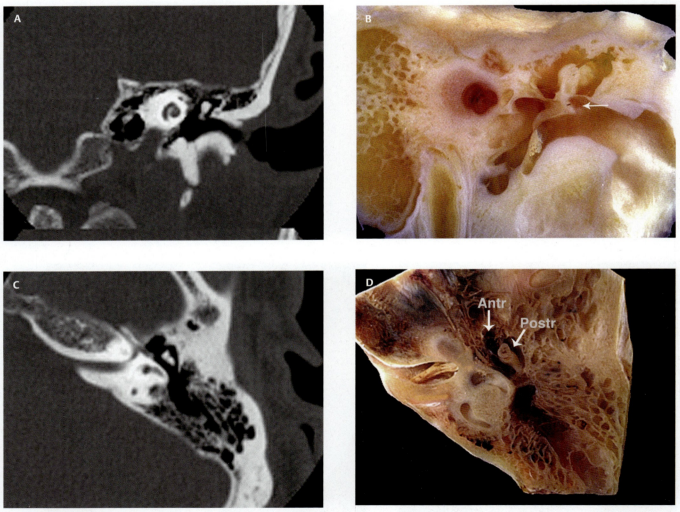

Fig. 1.8 The epitympanic spaces of von Troeltsch are formed by mucosal folds that separate the attic into anterior, posterior, and lateral compartments. These epitympanic spaces determine the pattern of growth of cholesteatoma. (**A**) Coronal CT image and (**B**) temporal bone sectioned in coronal plane, showing the lateral epitympanic, or Prussak's space (*horizontal arrow*). (**C**) Axial CT and (**D**) temporal bone sectioned in axial plane, showing anterior (*Antr*) and posterior (*Postr*) epitympanic spaces. (CT images and photos courtesy of Hiliary Brodie, MD).

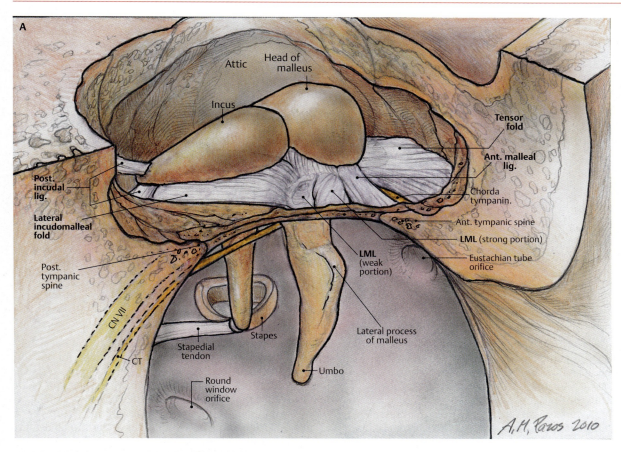

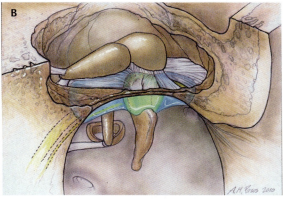

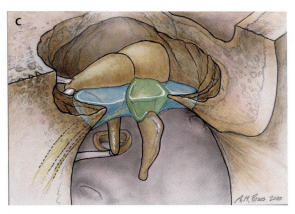

Fig. 1.9 **(A)** The epitympanic spaces described by von Troeltsch and Prussak, viewed from a lateral perspective, as they would appear to the surgeon, and from slightly above for artistic clarity. The epitympanic diaphragm divides the epitympanum into an upper and lower part. It consists, in the direction anterior to posterior, of the tensor fold, the anterior and lateral malleal ligamental folds (LML), the lateral incudomalleal fold, and the posterior incudal folds. **(B)** The lateral epitympanic (Prussak) space, shown in green, is bounded laterally by the Shrapnell membrane and medially by the neck of the malleus. The anterior and posterior epitympanic pouches, shown in blue, are separated from the Prussak space by thin membranes and are bounded superiorly by the lateral malleal fold, which forms part of the epitympanic membrane. The epitympanic diaphragm, consisting mainly of the lateral incudomalleal ligament and the duplicate mucosal membranes, separates the attic into upper and lower parts. The upper attic, which is superior to the malleus head and incus, communicates freely with the antrum through the aditus. **(C)** For clarity, the spaces are shown with the epitympanic diaphragm removed.

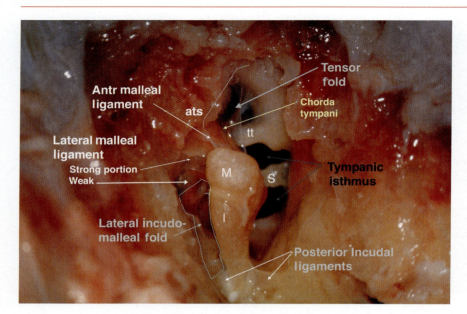

Fig. 1.10 Photograph of epitympanic dissection showing the structures that form the epitympanic diaphragm. This is a left ear, viewed from superiorly, looking down. (From Palva T, Ramsay H, Northrop C. Color Atlas of the Anatomy and Pathology of the Epitympanum. Basel, Switzerland: Karger; 2001. Reproduced courtesy of Professor Tauno Palva.)

Ramsay[15] recently wrote an excellent article that questioned Proctor's drawings, based on microdissection of 125 temporal bones, histologic study, and rereading of the original descriptions by the early anatomists. Palva's research group has described in detail the epitympanic diaphragm, which separates the large epitympanic compartments from the Prussak space and from the mesotympanum[15] (**Fig. 1.10**). It consists, in the direction anterior to posterior, of the tensor fold, the anterior and lateral malleal ligamental folds (the latter forms the roof of the Prussak space), the lateral incudomalleal fold, and the posterior incudal folds. The tensor fold and the lateral incudomalleal folds are thin duplicate folds, arising from a fusion of two advancing, opposing air sacs. The ligamental folds arise when the air sacs with the advancing epithelium, deriving from the eustachian tube, passes the preexisting ligaments. The anterior portion of the incudomalleal fold regularly turns inferiorly, uniting with the posterior portion of the roof of the Prussak space in the lateral malleal space. All compartments above the epitympanic diaphragm communicate with the antrum through the aditus.

The elegant publications of Palva's group[15,16] provide a clear explanation of the potential paths of the spread of cholesteatoma. Attic cholesteatoma that begins as a papillary ingrowth from the pars flaccida into the Prussak space will remain confined to this space if discovered early. Further extension occurs regularly via the posterior pouch, along the medial wall of the tympanic membrane into the superior mesotympanum (**Fig. 1.11**). Due to the relatively frequent membrane defects in the posterior malleal ligamental fold (36%) extension may also occur directly to the lower lateral

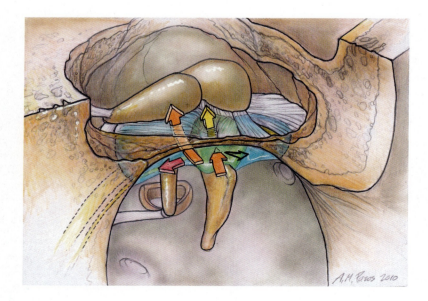

Fig. 1.11 Attic cholesteatomas that begin in the pars flaccida (*short orange arrow*) will remain confined to the Prussak space if discovered early. These cholesteatomas can enlarge into the posterior epitympanic space, via the posterior pouch (*red arrow*), or along the medial wall of the tympanic membrane into the superior mesotympanum (*green arrow*). Extension may also occur superiorly via a membrane defect (*long orange arrow*) or through the nonligamental weak portion of the roof of the Prussak space (*yellow arrow*), leading to the lateral malleal space; from there the routes are open to all compartments of the epitympanum.

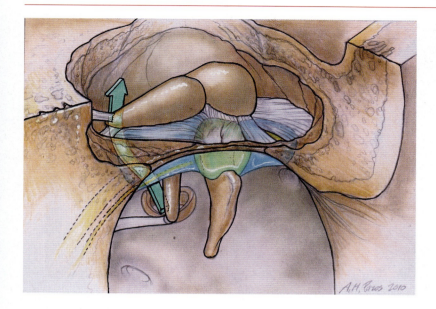

Fig. 1.12 Cholesteatoma that begins from the pars tensa can extend into the lower lateral attic, and via the tympanic isthmus, to all superior compartments of the epitympanum.

attic and to the superior mesotympanum. Extension superiorly can occur via a membrane defect or through the nonligamental weak portion of the roof of the Prussak space, leading to the lateral malleal space; from there the routes are open to all compartments of the epitympanum. Cholesteatoma that begins as a migrating ingrowth from the epidermal cells of the pars tensa can extend into the lower lateral attic and, via the tympanic isthmus, to all superior compartments of the epitympanum (**Fig. 1.12**). The supratubal recess, located in the anterior mesotympanum above the eustachian tube opening, can be invaded very rarely by a defect in the anterior membrane of the Prussak space, or in absence of the posterior pouch, from the lower lateral attic directly (**Fig. 1.13**).

These pathways of spread give rise to the patterns of growth of cholesteatoma that are encountered at surgery and have been classified as follows by Fraysse and others (**Fig. 1.14A–E**):

1. *Epitympanic (attic) cholesteatomas* arise from the pars flaccida and grow upward. These may be subdivided into *lateral epitympanic cholesteatomas*, if they involve only the Prussak space, *posterior epitympanic cholesteatomas*, if they grow medial to the incus to involve the posterior epitympanic space and mastoid, and *anterior epitympanic cholesteatomas* if they grow anteriorly to fill the space medial to the cog.

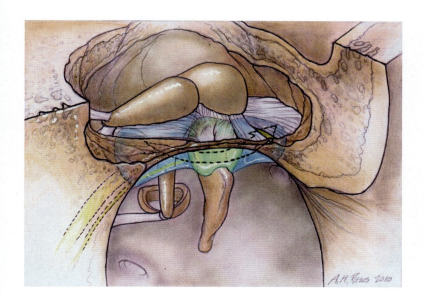

Fig. 1.13 An infrequent route of cholesteatoma to the supratubal recess. It starts from a defect in the anterior portion of the posterior malleal ligament and, due to marked indrawing of the posterior portion of the pars tensa, finds its way medial to the incus into the recess.

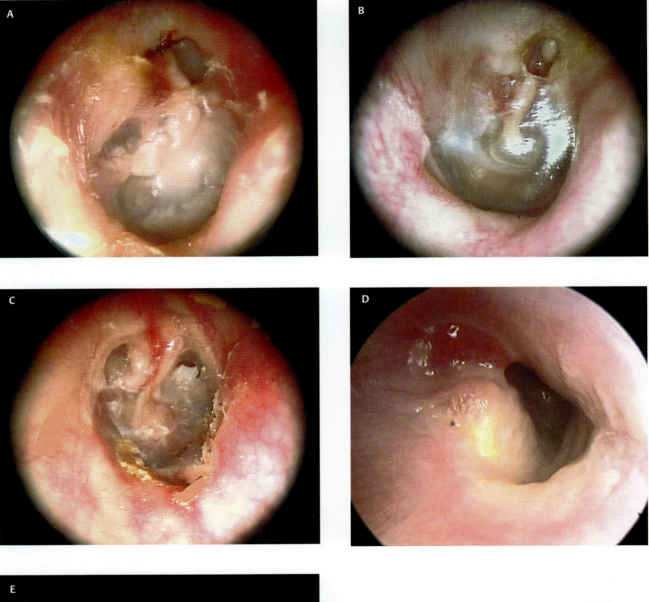

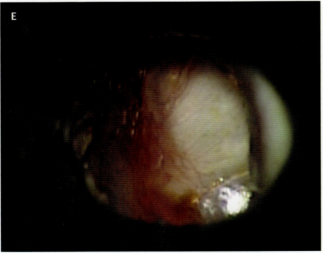

Fig. 1.14   The patterns of growth of cholesteatoma determine the surgical approach to their treatment. **(A)** Posterior epitympanic cholesteatomas begin in the pars flaccida and progress posteriorly, medial and lateral to the incus. **(B)** Anterior epitympanic cholesteatomas also begin in the pars flaccida but grow anterior to the head of the malleus. **(C)** Mesotympanic (middle ear) cholesteatomas begin in the posterior half of the pars tensa and grow medially, along the stapes and into the sinus tympani. **(D)** Holotympanic cholesteatomas can begin in the pars flaccida or pars tensa and grow to fill the middle ear, attic, and mastoid. **(E)** Congenital cholesteatomas form behind an intact tympanic membrane.

2. *Mesotympanic (middle ear) cholesteatomas* arise from the pars tensa and grow medially along the lenticular process and stapes superstructure. They may then grow upward toward the posterior epitympanum or backward into the sinus tympani, and they may fill the entire middle ear. (Sudhoff and Tos have further divided middle ear cholesteatomas into *sinus cholesteatomas*, posterosuperior quadrant retractions that fill the sinus tympani, and *tensa cholesteatomas*, which are diffuse retractions of the eardrum into the middle ear space[17]).

3. *Holotympanic cholesteatomas* involve the middle ear, epitympanum, and mastoid. These are epitympanic cholesteatomas that have grown down into the middle ear space, or middle ear cholesteatomas that have grown up into the attic.

4. *Congenital cholesteatomas* begin in the middle ear cleft, usually the anterosuperior quadrant attached to the tensor tympani tendon and processus cochleariformis, but may enlarge in all directions.

◆ Preoperative Assessment

Cholesteatoma occurs in adults and children of any age. Acquired cholesteatomas are far more common than congenital cholesteatomas. Acquired cholesteatomas are usually heralded by ear drainage, sometimes malodorous, and often persistent or recurrent despite treatment with antibiotic drops. Pain does not usually occur. Hearing loss is common but may not be reported by the patient and may go undetected in children. Tinnitus is rare. Vertigo is also uncommon and indicates the presence of labyrinthitis or labyrinthine fistula. Occasionally, the development of a suppurative complication (such as mastoiditis or even meningitis) is the first mode of presentation.

Physical Examination and Microscopy

The diagnosis of cholesteatoma is by physical examination, with imaging studies playing a confirmatory role. The physical examination should include otoscopy and otomicroscopy, and occasionally otoendoscopy. The benefits of microscopy include magnification, illumination (allowing one to see fluid or a sac through a translucent drum), binocular depth perception (useful for evaluating the extent of retraction pockets), and the ability to debride, suction, and probe. Under the microscope, the examiner can elevate crusts and suction away any pus or secretions. It is particularly important to inspect the attic, where cholesteatomas most commonly arise. Cholesteatoma will appear as a deep retraction pocket with purulent discharge or squamous epithelial debris. If the ear is acutely inflamed, a polyp may be present (**Fig. 1.15**), and careful debridement and cauterization will reveal the retraction pocket, yet to be described here. An attic polyp usually, but not always, signifies cholesteatoma; other forms of middle ear inflammation can occasionally cause polyps. A cholesteatoma sac may occasionally occur alongside a tympanic membrane perforation, so it is important to examine the attic even if a central perforation is present (**Fig. 1.16**).

The endoscope may supplement the view gained by microscopy. A short, zero-degree, 2.7 mm Hopkins rod–type telescope is ideal for otoendoscopy. The endoscope effectively places the examiner's eyeball inside the ear canal, allowing an unobstructed view of the entire drum. The endoscope may allow one to see deeply into a retraction pocket, to determine whether there is frank cholesteatoma. When mounted to a video capture system, it can produce an image that can be saved in the medical chart shown to the patient to bet-

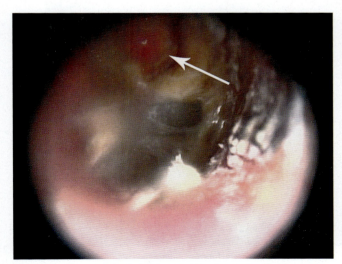

Fig. 1.15 Mucopurulent otorrhea and a polyp protruding from the attic (*arrow*) are typical physical findings of cholesteatoma.

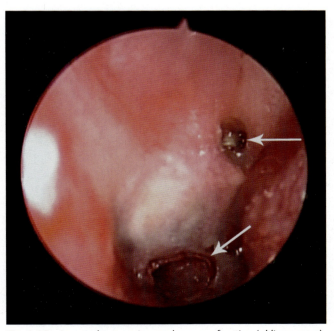

Fig. 1.16 A central tympanic membrane perforation (*oblique arrow*) in an ear with attic cholesteatoma (*horizontal arrow*).

ter explain the nature of the disease. The endoscope may be difficult to use in children who cannot hold still, and in the presence of pus or debris in the canal.

The physical examination should also include complete evaluation of the nose and throat, head and neck, lower cranial nerves, and gross assessment of hearing including tuning forks. The Weber test, in which a low-frequency tuning fork (256 or 512 Hz) is placed on a bony prominence in the center of the head, lateralizes toward the side of a conductive hearing loss and away from a sensorineural loss. The Rinne test compares bone conduction (on the mastoid bone) to air conduction (in front of the meatus) for each ear; in a negative Rinne, bone conduction is greater than air conduction, signifying a conductive hearing loss, and in a positive Rinne, air conduction is greater than bone, signifying either a sensorineural loss or normal hearing. Examination for nystagmus and fistula test should be performed in any patient reporting dizziness or imbalance. In the presence of acute labyrinthitis, nystagmus will be horizontal or horizontal-rotatory and unidirectional, with the quick component directed away from the side of the lesion, due to a hypofunctioning labyrinth. In the presence of a labyrinthine fistula, positive pressure in the ear canal produced with a cupped hand, pneumatic otoscope, or Politzer bag will elicit a sensation of vertigo, imbalance, or nausea, and deviation of the eyes. Traditionally, positive pressure would cause deviation of the eyes away from the test ear, and negative pressure will produce eye deviation toward the test ear. The direction of the eye deviation will actually depend on the exact location of the fistula, with the movement of the endolymph either toward or away from the cupula of the ampulated area of the semicircular canal.

The differential diagnosis of a chronic draining ear includes chronic suppurative otitis media (usually with tympanic membrane perforation), granulomatous otitis media, post-tympanostomy otorrhea, retained foreign body, acute otitis media with tympanic membrane rupture, acute coalescent mastoiditis, acute, chronic otitis externa, and granular myringitis. Drainage from a preexisting mastoidectomy cavity is usually from mucositis with granulation tissue or retained or trapped cholesteatoma, mastoid abscess, or occasionally osteitis. Malignant neoplasms should also be considered in elderly individuals with chronic relentless drainage, particularly if there is pain and an ulcerative mass in the ear canal. Malignant (or necrotizing) external otitis (MEO) occurs in elderly diabetics and immunocompromised individuals (AIDS, chemotherapy) and is characterized by deep, boring pain and chronic otorrhea, and the presence of granulation tissue at the bony–cartilaginous junction of the external canal on physical exam. The pathophysiology of MEO is osteomyelitis of the tympanic bone, which can spread to involve the entire skull base. The bacteriology is usually *Pseudomonas*, and the treatment usually involves a quinolone antibiotic, although antibiotic resistance is common, so culture and sensitivity are advisable.

The presence of polyp (raised infected granulation tissue) usually signifies cholesteatoma, but polyps may also occur in the presence of chronic otitis externa, malignant otitis externa, retained ventilating tubes, and neoplasms of the ear canal. Benign neoplasms of the ear canal include pleomorphic adenoma and ceruminous adenoma; malignancies include adenoid cystic carcinoma, squamous cell carcinoma, and basal cell carcinoma of meatal or conchal origin.

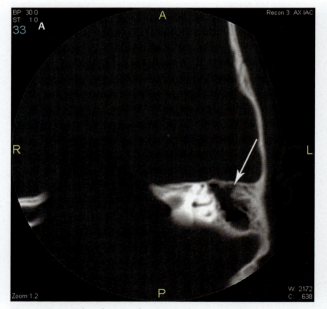 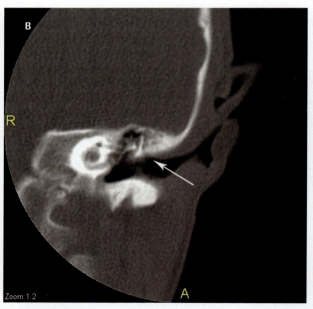

Fig. 1.17 Axial and coronal computed tomographic scans of attic cholesteatoma with extension to the mastoid antrum. **(A)** The axial scan shows demineralization ("coalescence") of the trabecular bone around the antrum (*arrow*). **(B)** The coronal scan shows soft tissue in the attic and superior middle ear space with blunting of the scutum (*arrow*). The disease envelops the malleus head.

The Role of Imaging

CT scanning is often performed in patients with cholesteatoma. Whether CT should be obtained routinely or selectively remains a matter of debate, but most surgeons would agree that a preoperative CT scan is nice to have. This is especially true in the patient with dizziness, sensorineural hearing loss, headache, or facial nerve palsy or twitching. Except in very few instances, the diagnosis of cholesteatoma can be made clinically on otomicroscopy; thus CT is not necessary to make the diagnosis. The radiologic hallmarks of cholesteatoma are soft tissue in the attic with bone erosion of the scutum (lateral epitympanic wall), mastoid air cells, or ossicles (**Fig. 1.17A,B**). There are infrequent cases in which an acquired cholesteatoma will be identified on CT but not on physical exam, either because the mouth of the cholesteatoma sac has become obliterated by inflammatory swelling or because polypoid granulation tissue limits examination of the attic.

The main value of CT is for preoperative planning—to determine the *size* of the mastoid cavity, the *extent of disease*, and the presence of potential *complications*. CT provides an anatomical roadmap that can be used at surgery.

Mastoid size can be classified as developed, diploic, or sclerotic (**Fig. 1.18A–C**), and the degree of cellularity is an important factor in deciding how the canal wall is dealt with at surgery. Mastoid air cell development begins in early childhood and is inhibited by the presence of inflammatory disease. *Sclerotic* mastoids are poorly developed, and the bone appears dense (like the sclera of the eye). Surgery can be difficult in a sclerotic mastoid because of the absence of landmarks, but the resulting surgical cavity can be expected to be small. Therefore canal wall down surgery in a sclerotic mastoid usually results in good surgical exposure and a small resultant cavity. *Diploic* mastoids are marrow filled. There are also few air cells, but the extent of pneumatization can be variable. Marrow bone bleeds during drilling. *Developed* (or "pneumatized") mastoids can have any degree of cellularity (the term *pneumatized* is more commonly used but is strictly speaking incorrect, if there is extensive cellularity but the cells are filled with soft tissue rather than air). An extensively developed mastoid will

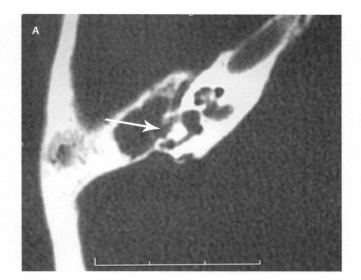

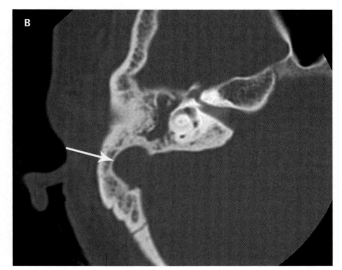

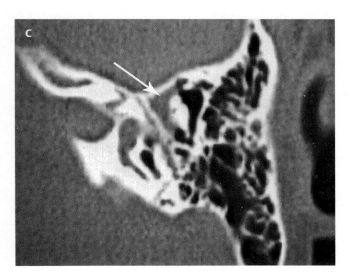

Fig. 1.18 Computed tomography is useful for determining mastoid size and anatomy, extent of disease, and presence of complications, such as lateral semicircular canal fistula. **(A)** Sclerotic mastoid with lateral semicircular canal fistula (*arrow*). **(B)** Diploic mastoid, which has poor cellularity and some marrow spaces, with forward-lying sigmoid sinus (*arrow*). **(C)** Well developed mastoid with extensive pneumatization, cholesteatoma located medial to ossicles (*arrow*).

result in a large cavity if the canal wall is taken down, and it may be difficult to manage postoperatively.

CT can also help determine the extent of disease. Cholesteatomas confined to the attic or middle ear might be managed differently than cholesteatomas that fill the entire mastoid. In cases confined to the attic, the presence or absence of disease in the anterior epitympanic space might be a deciding factor in leaving or removing the posterior canal wall. The height of the epitympanum, the distance between the superior bony canal wall and the tegmen tympani, determines the surgical exposure that can be obtained through a transmastoid atticotomy. Disease confined to the lateral epitympanic space (the Prussak space) may be approached through a limited atticotomy. CT can underestimate the extent of disease, however, in those cases in which the cholesteatoma sac is empty (ie, not filled with debris) (**Fig. 1.19**).

CT is also useful for detecting impending complications, such as erosion of the lateral semicircular canal, the fallopian canal, or the tegmen. Surgical injury can be prevented if there is a very forward-lying sigmoid sinus or high jugular bulb in the middle ear. In cases with existing preoperative complications, such as subperiosteal or Bezold abscess, vertigo with suspected fistula, sensorineural hearing loss, facial nerve paresis, retrobulbar headache, or meningeal signs, preoperative CT scanning should be considered mandatory. Magnetic resonance imaging (MRI) may also be helpful when intracranial complications or abscess are suspected clinically.

The Wet Ear

If the ear is draining at the time of presentation, measures should be taken to clear up the drainage, both to enable proper inspection for preoperative diagnosis and to facilitate surgery. Sometimes, however, the infection will prove to be refractory, and the drainage will not resolve until the cholesteatoma is removed.

Careful suction-debridement can be done under a microscope, removing the pus and stagnant debris down to the plane of the drum. Patients are usually cooperative with this procedure as long as the examiner avoids touching the canal wall skin, which can be sensitive. In children, suctioning can usually be achieved with calm reassurance and the assistance of the parent. The majority of cholesteatomas arise from the attic, so it is beneficial to carefully inspect this area and remove any crusts.

When a polyp is present, it can often be removed, which facilitates examination of the attic and also helps resolve the drainage. Excision of the polyp can be accomplished by lifting it with a suction, cauterizing the stalk with silver nitrate, and gently debriding the tissue with suction or alligator forceps. This is a helpful maneuver, both to allow a complete view of the attic and to remove the source of drainage. Polyps are insensate, and so debridement is feasible in all but young children. Bleeding may occur, which may be disturbing to the parent but is not dangerous to the patient.

In an actively draining ear, it is useful to culture the discharge to identify the causative organism and select an effective antibiotic. The most common organisms are *Pseudomonas* sp. and other gram-negative bacilli, *Staphylococcus aureus*, and (rarely) fungi and anaerobes.

Applying boric acid powder with an atomizer or powder blower can help dry the ear by absorption, and acidifying the medium has a bactericidal and fungicidal effect too. Other topical medicaments have also been used successfully. Patients should continue antibacterial ear drops at home, such as a quinolone antibiotic drop (often with a steroid to decrease the inflammatory response) or 2% acetic acid solution. If long-term (> 2 to 3 weeks) administration of eardrops is necessary, a nonantibiotic solution is preferred to avoid fungal overgrowth. Suctioning in the office at weekly or biweekly intervals will usually result in a dry ear before surgery is undertaken.

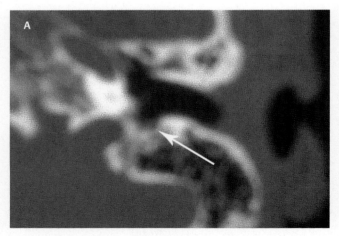
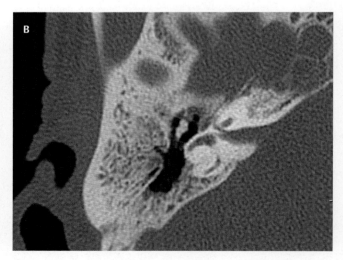

Fig. 1.19 Computed tomography can underestimate the extent of disease. **(A)** This scan is normal except for a small rim of soft tissue in the sinus tympani (*arrow*); at surgery, the child had an invasive middle ear cholesteatoma. **(B)** This scan shows a small area of soft tissue in the antrum; at surgery the disease filled the entire mastoid, but the sac was mostly empty.

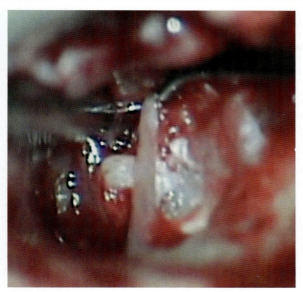

Fig. 1.20 Preserving the chorda tympani.

◆ Preoperative Counseling

Expected Results: Risks, Benefits, and Alternatives

The goals of surgery are to remove the disease completely, preserve or restore hearing, and minimize the chance of recurrence. The most common risks of cholesteatoma surgery are hearing loss, recurrence of the disease, and the need for more than one operation. Less common risks of surgery include recurrent infection or drainage, dysgeusia (from involvement of the chorda tympani nerve—**Fig. 1.20**), stenosis of the external auditory canal, dizziness or imbalance, tinnitus, bleeding, and facial nerve paralysis. There are in effect no alternatives to surgery. The presence of cholesteatoma mandates surgical treatment, and, although this is rarely urgent, it is not optional because there are no medical alternatives to removing the disease. Patients with concurrent medical problems in whom surgery or anesthesia is contraindicated should have their infection managed medically in the office and be told to follow strict dry ear precautions.

Risk of Recurrence

The biological fact that makes cholesteatoma surgery daunting is that the disease has a tendency to recur, even in the hands of the most experienced surgeon. This is true regardless of whether canal wall up or canal wall down technique is used (although recurrence is less common in canal wall down surgery). The rate of recurrence tends to be higher in children than in adults. The regrowth of cholesteatoma can occur in two ways: true *recurrence* is the redevelopment of cholesteatoma in the surgical cavity from a new retraction pocket; *residual* cholesteatoma is disease left behind by the surgeon.

Patients need to be informed that cholesteatoma can recur after the most thorough operation. This mandates regular clin-

ical follow-up, usually every 6 months for several years after the surgery. It also raises the possibility of needing more than one operation. In some situations, a two-stage approach is planned from the outset; this issue is discussed in Chapter 8.

Need for Additional Surgery

The surgeon attempts to create a dry, safe ear without cholesteatoma. This can often, but not always, be achieved in a single operation. Reasons for second (and sometimes even third) surgical procedures include residual or recurrent cholesteatoma, hearing loss requiring ossicular reconstruction, meatal stenosis, chronic mastoid mucositis requiring revision mastoidectomy ± skin grafting or cavity obliteration, tympanic membrane perforation requiring tympanoplasty, tympanic membrane collapse requiring myringotomy tube or cartilage tympanoplasty or both, and occasionally for the treatment of complications.

◆ Postoperative Care

Cholesteatoma surgery can usually be done on an outpatient basis. Patients are given a prescription of pain medication and are told to avoid water in the ear, avoid straining and heavy lifting, and avoid blowing the nose vigorously. The first follow-up visit is scheduled for 7 to 10 days after surgery.

There are postoperative risks to those patients who are using sleep apnea positive pressure devices. In those patients, we use additional packing in the eustachian tube during surgery and ask them to limit the use in the immediate postoperative time if medically feasible.

There are many variations on the further postop routine, guided mainly by the surgeon's preference. We instruct the patient to remove the mastoid dressing (a cotton gauze fluff held in place with a stretch-gauze roll) on the first postop day and leave the wound open to air. The postauricular incision can be dressed with bacitracin ointment twice a day. A clean cotton ball can be placed in the meatus and changed once a day, or more often if there is bleeding. Patients are told to call if there is fever, increasing postauricular swelling, or pus from the meatus or wound. Antibiotics are not generally given.

At the first visit (7 to 10 days postoperative), we remove the outer packing to the tympanic membrane reconstruction site. The postauricular area is cleaned and then dressed with an antibiotic ointment. We use a subcuticular closure in most cases (chromic or Monocryl, Ethicon, Inc, Somerville, NJ) so that suture removal is not needed. Patients are started on antibiotic eardrops (ofloxacin or ciprofloxacin, with steroids if much inflammatory reaction is present), and seen again at 2- or 3-week intervals until the ear is healed. Unresorbed gelatin packing is removed with suction or forceps at the second visit. If a meatoplasty was performed, granulations are managed with a light application of silver nitrate. An audiogram is obtained when the eardrum is fully healed, at around 6 to 12 weeks. Regular surveillance follow-up is then scheduled at 6-month intervals.

References

1. Schuknecht HF. Pathology of the Ear. 2nd ed. Philadelphia, PA: Lea & Febiger; 1993:204–206
2. Semaan MT, Megerian CA. The pathophysiology of cholesteatoma. Otolaryngol Clin North Am 2006;39(6):1143–1159
3. Olszewska E, Wagner M, Bernal-Sprekelsen M, et al. Etiopathogenesis of cholesteatoma. Eur Arch Otorhinolaryngol 2004;261(1):6–24
4. Sudhoff H, Bujía J, Borkowshi G, et al. Basement membrane in middle ear cholesteatoma: immunohistochemical and ultrastructural observations. Ann Otol Rhinol Laryngol 1996;105(10):804–810
5. Michaels L. Origin of congenital cholesteatoma from a normally occurring epidermoid rest in the developing middle ear. Int J Pediatr Otorhinolaryngol 1988;15(1):51–65
6. Abramson M. Collagenolytic activity in middle ear cholesteatoma. Ann Otol Rhinol Laryngol 1969;78(1):112–124
7. Abramson M, Moriyama H, Huang CC. Histology, pathogenesis, and treatment of cholesteatoma. Ann Otol Rhinol Laryngol Suppl 1984;112:125–128
8. Moriyama H, Honda Y, Huang CC, Abramson M. Bone resorption in cholesteatoma: epithelial-mesenchymal cell interaction and collagenase production. Laryngoscope 1987;97(7 Pt 1):854–859
9. Jung JY, Chole RA. Bone resorption in chronic otitis media: the role of the osteoclast. ORL J Otorhinolaryngol Relat Spec 2002;64(2):95–107
10. Von Troeltsch A. Lehrbuch der Ohrenheilkunde mit Einschluss der anatomie des Ohres. 7th ed. Leipzig, Germany: FCW Vogel; 1881
11. Hammar JA. Studien uber die Entwicklung des Vorderdans und eineger angrandzenden Organe. Arch Mikroskop Anat 1902;59:471–628
12. Prussak A. Zur Anatomie des menschlichen Trommelfells. Arch Ohernheilkd 1867;3:255–278
13. Siebenmann F. Miggelohr und Labyrinth. In: Bardeleben K von, ed. Handbuch der Anatomie des Menschen. Vol 5. Jena, Germany: Fischer; 1897:244–287
14. Proctor B. The development of the middle ear spaces and their surgical significance. J Laryngol Otol 1964;78:631–648
15. Palva T, Ramsay H, Northrop C. Color Atlas of the Anatomy and Pathology of the Epitympanum. Basel, Switzerland: Karger; 2001
16. Palva T, Ramsay H. Aeration of Prussak's space is independent of the supradiaphragmatic epitympanic compartments. Otol Neurotol 2007;28(2):264–268
17. Sudhoff H, Tos M. Pathogenesis of sinus cholesteatoma. Eur Arch Otorhinolaryngol 2007;264:1137–1143

2
Tympanoplasty: Indications and Technique

Today the goal of successful tympanoplasty is to create a mobile tympanic membrane or graft with an aerated mucosal-lined middle ear space and a sound-conducting mechanism between the mobile membrane and the inner ear fluids. A review of the literature reveals that many techniques have been developed and employed successfully, and there is a rich history of the evolution of techniques to produce this end. With this review the authors hope to describe a brief history of the evolution of the over–under tympanoplasty, with indications and technical aspects of the technique.

◆ Tympanic Membrane and Middle Ear Cleft

Embryologically, the tympanic membrane is derived from the fusion of the ectodermal meatal plugs from the first branchial cleft and the endodermally derived first branchial pouch (tubotympanic recess). The tympanic membrane and middle ear cavity make up the area of contact between these two structures. The tympanic membrane separates the delicate middle and inner ear structures from the external environment. It measures ~10 mm in diameter and is conically shaped with the apex of the cone at the umbo.

Histologically, the tympanic membrane has three layers. This structure contains an outer ectodermal layer composed of keratinizing squamous epithelium, a middle mesodermal fibrous layer, and an inner endodermal mucosal layer. The outer epidermal layer is composed of stratum corneum, granulosum, spinosum, and basale. This layer has cell growth and migratory properties responsible for the self-cleaning and replacement function of the tympanic membrane.[1,2] Studies have demonstrated the presence of epidermal growth factor and fibroblast growth factor, which are thought to promote healing of membrane perforations and contribute to the success of tympanoplasty procedures.[3]

The mesodermal fibrous layer is the intermediate layer or the lamina propria. There are different compositions depending on the location along the tympanic membrane.[4] In the pars tensa the lamina propria has a subepidermal loose connective tissue layer containing the internal blood vessels and nerves and a fibrous layer made of outer radial and inner circular fibers. These fibers are made of collagen. This should contribute to the vibratory functions of the tympanic membrane.[5,6] The pars flaccida or Shrapnell membrane has elastic fibers and accounts for the flaccidity of this variably sized area.[4]

There are two major blood supplies of the tympanic membrane. An external plexus from the tympanic branch of the deep auricular artery sends large manubrial branches along the Shrapnell membrane and the manubrium and numerous radial branches into the tympanic membrane from along its circumference.[7] The malleal artery is the major blood supply of the posterior half of the tympanic membrane, which is better perfused than the anterior half.[8] The anterior half is supplied from smaller radial branches that enter around the annulus derived from the internal plexus from the stylomastoid branch of the postauricular artery.[7]

The middle ear (*mesotympanum*) is the air-containing space that is bounded laterally by the tympanic membrane. The medial wall of the middle ear is formed by the promontory, which is the lateral bony wall of the cochlea, and which is covered by a thin layer of mucosa (mainly nonkeratinizing low cuboidal epithelium or ciliated columnar epithelium in places). The anterior portion of the middle ear, termed the *protympanum*, contains the bony opening of the eustachian tube. The inferior middle ear (*hypotympanum*) contains air cells; posteriorly the jugular bulb may be present. The superior middle ear is confluent with the *epitympanum*, or attic, which contains the head of the malleus and body of the incus. Posteriorly, the middle ear is bounded by the bony ear canal, the mastoid segment of the facial nerve, and the pneumatized cell tract called the facial recess. Inferior to the facial nerve is a space named the *sinus tympani*, important in cholesteatoma surgery because it is a frequent site for recurrence.

The middle ear contains the ossicles—malleus, incus, and stapes—and the tympanic segment of the facial nerve, chorda tympani nerve, tensor tympani, and stapedius muscles. The mucosa of the middle ear envelops the ossicles like a mesentery and forms a very fine layer that partitions the air-containing space and determines the direction that disease may grow (as discussed in Chapter 1).

The middle ear contains the ossicular chain with its ligaments and the tendons of the tensor tympani and stapedius muscles. The attic or epitympanum is almost completely separated from the mesotympanum by the ossicles and their folds except for two small but constant spaces. The Prussak space is bounded superiorly by the lateral malleolar fold arising from the junction of the malleus head and neck and radiates out to insert on the entire bony rim of the notch of Rivinus.

◆ Historical Review

The tympanoplasty operation is a surgical procedure to eradicate disease in the middle ear and to reconstruct the hearing mechanism, with or without mastoid surgery, with or without tympanic membrane grafting. This was defined by the American Academy of Ophthalmology and Otolaryngology's Committee on Conservation of Hearing in 1964.[9] Hippocrates recognized that "acute pain of the ear, with continued strong fevers, is to be dreaded, for there is danger that the man may become delirious and die."[10] Early surgery for the draining ear was basically a mastoid operation and was life saving. The first attempt to repair a tympanic membrane was performed in 1640 when Banzer used a pig's bladder stretched across an ivory tube and placed in the ear, which gave temporary hearing improvement.[11] In 1853, Toynbee placed a rubber disc attached to a silver wire over a perforation with hearing improvement.[12] In 1877, Blake placed a paper patch over a perforation, and in many patients a hearing improvement was noted.[13]

The concept of tympanoplasty is credited to Berthold who in 1878 was thought to have performed the first true tympanoplasty. His technique involved deepithelializing the tympanic membrane by applying plaster against the membrane for 3 days, removing the epithelium, and then placing a skin graft over the defect.[14] The "modern era" of tympanoplasty occurred in the 1950s because of many developments in antibiotics, instrumentation, and the operating microscope.

Following the introduction of tympanoplasty by Wullstein and Zollner in the early 1950s, all surgeries used an overlay graft.[15,16] Wullstein's paper, "Tympanoplasty as an Operation to Improve Hearing in Chronic Otitis Media and Its Results" set the stage for this operation to improve hearing and protect the middle ear from the outside environment. At that time, this consisted of full-thickness and split-thickness skin grafts. By the end of the decade, graft eczema, desquamation and poor long-term take rate had prompted many surgeons to seed alternate grafting materials and techniques.[17] In 1956, Sooy had reported the use of canal skin pedicle graft to close marginal perforations.[18] In 1958, House and Sheehy and Plester working independently began using canal skin as a free overlay graft.[19,20] Shea, Austin, and Tabb working independently in 1959 employed vein as an undersurface graft to repair tympanic membrane perforations.[21-23] The vein graft tended to atrophy over a few months and occasionally

reperforated. In 1961 Storrs described the first undersurface fascia technique to be used in this country.[24] With the use of connective tissue most of the problems incurred with free skin grafts were eliminated. The first successful use of homograft tympanic membrane in this country was by Ned Chalat in 1964.[25] His experience was reported in the Harper Hospital Bulletin and went unnoticed for several years. Many authors reported promising results with this technique in 1968 by House and Glasscock, and soon to be followed by Perkins, Smith, and Wehrs.[26-29] With this technique procurement and sterilization of the donor material have been problematic. Over the years surgeons have used various living or homograft grafting materials already mentioned, including loose areolar connective tissue, perichondrium, cartilage, fat, and periostium.[30,31]

Fascia has been the preferred material because of the internal structure of this material and because of the plentiful amount in the operative field. The high success rate of this material probably resides in the internal structure of collagen and mucopolysaccharides. It is interesting to note that both collagen and mucopolysaccharides have been implicated as playing a critical role in wound healing. Collagen is felt to contribute to wound tensile strength, and there is evidence that the chemically and biologically complex mucopolysaccharides play a positive role in the healing process, attracting fibroblasts into the wound area through chemotaxis.[32]

◆ Conditions of the Middle Ear in Tympanoplasty Surgery

Perforated Eardrum That Is Dry

With a dry perforated eardrum the surgeon needs to assess the size, location, and middle ear spacing (retracted ossicular chain, narrow middle ear cleft, lateral promontory, or high jugular bulb). Depending on the particular situation encountered, one may then choose underlay, overlay or over–under tympanoplasty technique (**Fig. 2.1**).

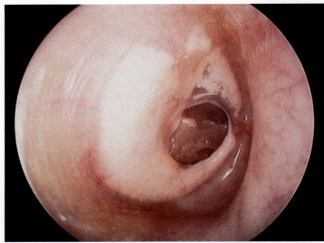

Fig. 2.1 Tympanic membrane perforation with tympanosclerosis.

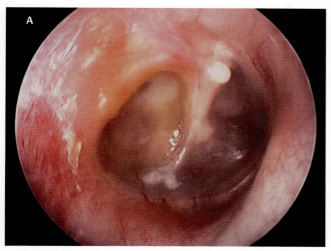
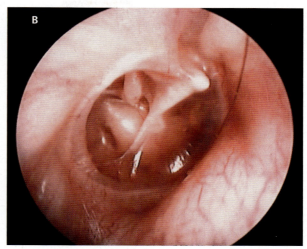

Fig. 2.2 (A) Chronic suppurative otitis media. (B) Previous ear, treated with oral and topical antibiotics.

Perforated Eardrum with Chronic Suppurative Otitis Media

With chronic suppurative otitis media (CSOM) one tries to dry the drainage if possible with general medical procedures such as topical and oral antibiotics, improvement of eustachian tube dysfunction, or allergy management. In some patients the drainage may not be controlled prior to surgery. The principles outlined earlier are followed, with the possible addition of an aerating mastoidectomy in a select patient group (**Fig. 2.2A,B**).

Perforated Eardrum Secondary to Cholesteatoma

One must determine whether the perforation caused by the cholesteatoma is confined to the middle ear or extends into the epitympanic space or mastoid (**Fig. 2.3**).

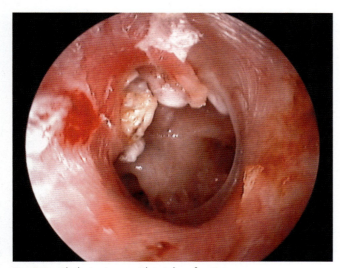

Fig. 2.3 Cholesteatoma with total perforation.

◆ Techniques

Evolution of Techniques

A review of the literature reveals that many techniques have been developed and employed successfully. Tympanoplasty techniques have employed approaches such as transcanal, endaural, or postauricular. The grafts have been placed over and under the tympanic membrane or the malleus, and the biological material used has been full-thickness skin, partial-thickness skin, fascia, perichondrium, cartilage, and periosteum. We will describe the various techniques and approaches commonly used in the past and a personal evolution of technique for the majority of surgery utilizing the over–under tympanoplasty.

Underlay (Undersurface) Technique

The underlay or undersurface technique employs the use of grafting material medial or under the remnant tympanic membrane typically under the malleus when the perforation extends to that area. The free edges of the perforation are prepared using a right-angled hook, and in some instances, a fine scissors is used to resect the perforation margins. The intent is to separate the outer cutaneous layer from underturned epithelium or separate the inner mucosal layer from the external tympanic membrane epithelium. This develops a fresh edge for healing. This technique, originally described by Shea in 1957, was used initially for iatrogenic tympanic membrane perforations caused at the time of middle ear surgery.[28] Austin and Shea in 1961 published their combined experience with this technique stating that vein was an ideal material because it did not substitute for the missing squamous layer of the drum, but as a replacement for the fibrous layer across which normal epithelium will grow.[33] The great hardiness of the vein as a free graft was also thought to be desirable. Their approach began as a transcanal or transmeatal procedure. The postauricular approach was used as a surgeon's decision at the time of surgery. Long-term results with vein proved to be fraught with atrophy over a few months and occasionally re-perforated. These results were improved with the use of fascia, loose areolar connective tissue, or perichondrial tissue and have been the preferred material over the past 40 years (**Fig. 2.4A–D**).

Overlay Technique

The overlay technique as practiced in the 1960s and occasionally used today, consisted of accessing the drum head through the surgeon's preferred incision. The epithelium of the surface of the drum was removed, a fascia graft was placed on the perforation, and the ear was packed with various materials. Sheehy and Glasscock replaced the pedicled canal skin grafts earlier described by authors with temporalis fascia overlay grafts.[34] After comparing cases of canal skin and fascia grafts the following conclusions were made: (1) fascia grafts (97.5% take rate) were generally superior to canal skin grafts (91.8% take rate); (2) fascia grafts were also superior (91%) to canal skin grafts (70%) in closing total perforations; and (3) fascia was an excellent material to close ears that were draining at the time of surgery as evidenced by higher success rate (98%) than dry perforations using canal skin.

This technique was to be performed from the postauricular approach. Once the vascular strip incision is dissected out of the ear canal, it is held anteriorly with the retractor. The medial superior, anterior, and inferior canal wall skin is incised near the bony–cartilaginous junction and then carefully elevated medially to the annulus. The entire cuff of skin is then cut free leaving the annulus in its physiological position. This skin is then removed from the operative site and placed into saline for the duration of the case. Canal wall widening is performed with a small drill as needed to visualize the anterior portion of the annulus, and marked manipulation of anterior ear canal wall skin and drilling of the bone is necessary. The squamous layer of the tympanic membrane remnant, fascia placed in the physiological position of the drum, and then

the ear canal skin replaced over the fascia. The vascular strip is replaced, and the ear canal is packed with pledgets of absorbable gelatin sponge moistened in an antibiotic solution. With this technique, there is obvious marked bony and soft tissue dissection necessary, and ear drum blunting common, with frequent conductive hearing loss.

Indications for Over–Under Tympanoplasty

By combining the benefits of both techniques, the over–under tympanoplasty has become the preferred technique for various approaches to tympanoplasty.[35-37] This technique places the tympanic membrane fascia graft lateral to the malleus but medial to the remnant of tympanic membrane and fibrous annulus and medial to the bony annulus anteriorly and inferiorly. This allows excellent exposure to the anterior middle ear space and prevents medialization of the graft to the promontory. Ossicular reconstruction may be placed directly to the underside of the malleus. Over–under tympanoplasty has become a preferred technique for perforations that abut the malleus (**Fig. 2.5**), large or near total perforations, cases of significant malleus retraction (making the classic underlay technique impractical) (**Fig. 2.6**), significant anterior tympanosclerosis, or anterior middle ear cholesteatoma (**Table 2.1**).

The over–under tympanoplasty has been popularized recently as a technique for certain perforations.

Surgical Technique of Over–Under Tympanoplasty

Previous authors have demonstrated the technique of placing a graft lateral to the malleus but medial to the remnant of the tympanic membrane. As early as 1972, Austin stated that the graft may be secured either over or under the malleus tip, depending on the ease of positioning, and then some of the skin covering the malleus is dissected and replaced on the graft surface.[38] Glasscock, Wehrs, and Hough also made similar inferences when describing underlay grafting

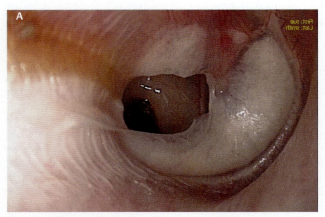
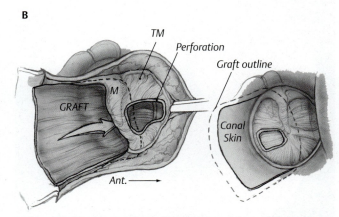

Fig. 2.4 **(A)** Tympanic membrane perforation with adequate middle ear space for underlay tympanoplasty. **(B)** Exposure of the middle ear after trimming the margins of perforation.

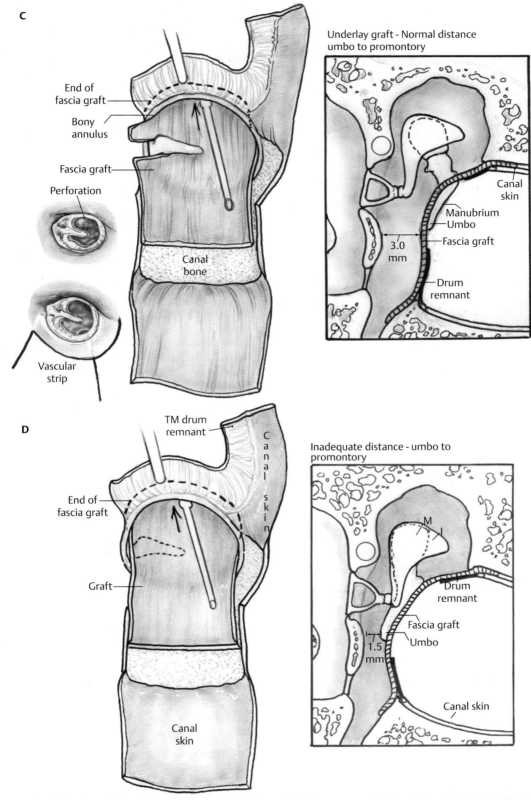

C

End of fascia graft

Bony annulus

Fascia graft

Perforation

Vascular strip

Canal bone

Underlay graft - Normal distance umbo to promontory

Canal skin

Manubrium

Umbo

Fascia graft

3.0 mm

Drum remnant

D

TM drum remnant

Canal skin

End of fascia graft

Graft

Canal skin

Inadequate distance - umbo to promontory

M

I

Drum remnant

Fascia graft

Umbo

1.5 mm

Canal skin

Fig. 2.4 (*Continued*) **(C)** Fascia graft placed under malleus and onto posterior bony ear canal wall, underlay technique. **(D)** Tympanic membrane and medial ear canal wall skin replaced onto the fascia graft.

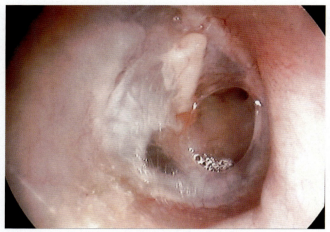

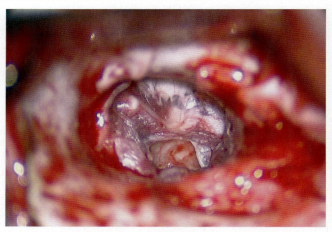

Fig. 2.5 Tympanic membrane perforation that abuts the malleus in the retraced middle ear space.

Fig. 2.6 Tympanic membrane with malleus retraction.

in particular situations, usually with significant retraction of the malleus, large perforations, or anterior middle ear disease.[39–41] In 2001, Kartush et al presented their results with this technique, including excellent long-term results for closure of perforations, hearing improvement or stabilization, and low incidence of complications.[42] The authors used this with and without mastoidectomy and with and without ossicular reconstruction.

Postauricular over–under tympanoplasty technique is begun with appropriate preoperative decisions common in all tympanoplasty surgery previously described elsewhere.

Surgical Preparation

Most patients will undergo general anesthesia with endotracheal intubation for this type of surgery. After anesthesia is secured, the patient is turned 180 degrees. The surgeon will sit at the surgical side of the patient, with the scrub nurse across the patient from the surgeon. An area of hair is removed from around the ear for ~2 cm above and behind the auricle. The natural oils of the skin are removed with alcohol solution or acetone, adherence material is placed on the edges of the prepped area, and plastic drapes are placed to the shaved area to hold the hair out of the field. The ear is injected with lidocaine-HCl 1% with 1:100,000 epinephrine in a subdermal plane at the postauricular incision site and a four-quadrant external ear location. A cotton ball is placed in the ear canal (to keep the scrub solution from the middle ear space), and the ear is then washed with an iodine solution, the solution being kept in contact with the ear for ~6 minutes. The ear is then dried from the solution by the

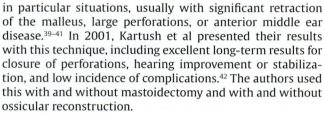

Table 2.1 Over–Under Tympanoplasty Highpoints

Fascia
Periostium incised and elevated
Fibrous tissue removed from umbo
Graft placement

scrub nurse, the ear is folded forward, and a plastic drape attached to a waterproof barrier is applied.

The drill cord, irrigation and suction tubes, and cautery lines are wrapped in a towel and placed and secured to the top of the drape over the patient. A second pouch is made to hold the drill handpiece, suction tips, and cautery devices. This prevents the lines from tangling or falling off the surgical field.

The surgeon then cuts the drape directly over the surgical site. A wet sponge is used to clean the external ear of any dried iodine solution, and then the ear is dried.

The ear canal is then suctioned free from any ear canal debris or iodine solution. The vascular strip area is examined and then injected with the same lidocaine–epinephrine solution at the boney cartilaginous junction site. The surgeon is to observe blanching of the skin of the vascular strip skin. The ear is then irrigated with sterile saline solution to further debride and clean the ear canal and examine the tympanic membrane pathology.

Incisions

The auricle is then held by the right-handed surgeon with the left hand, pulling the ear forward and laterally. The incision is made with a No. 15 blade ~5 mm behind the postauricular fold. Once the area of the loose areolar tissue overlying the temporalis fascia is seen, this bloodless plane is carried to the mastoid tip inferiorly. The nurse holds the auricle, and bleeding points are controlled with an electrocautery. A self-retaining retractor is then placed.

Harvesting Fascia

The scrub nurse holds the superior edge of the wound laterally with a small retractor to help visualize the fascia. We attempt to harvest true fascia for the reasons previously mentioned. Fascia of the temporalis muscle posteriorly is ideal because anteriorly the fascia thickens and occasionally splits with adipose tissue interposed. An incision is made in the fascia superior and parallel to the linea temporalis, and then a delicate iris scissors is used to harvest simply the

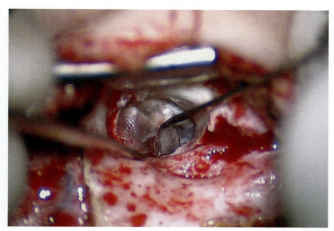

Fig. 2.7   Beaver blade tympanomeatal cut.

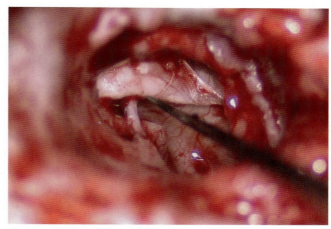

Fig. 2.8   Exposing the middle ear.

fascia without areolar tissue laterally or muscle tissue medially. For a subtotal perforation the graft is ~10 by 15 mm and for larger perforations a 15 by 20 mm graft is harvested. The graft is then placed on a Teflon block, cleaned of any areolar or muscle tissue, and then straightened on the block. The block is then placed onto the scrub nurse's back table where a lamp is placed near the graft to dehydrate the graft. Once the graft is dehydrated the lamp is turned off to prevent excessive drying of the graft.

Exposing the Ear Canal and Middle Ear

The area of the linea temporalis is palpated, and then an incision is made along this line between the temporalis muscle and the ear canal. A "T" incision is made through the tissue overlying the mastoid to the mastoid tip. A Lempert periosteal elevator is used to expose the mastoid bone, and the spine of Henle is visualized.

The self-retaining retractor is placed in this deeper plane. Now with the use of the operating microscope, a smaller periosteal elevator in the surgeon's right hand and a fine 20-gauge suction in the left hand are used to elevate the soft tissue of the bony external ear canal. Care is taken not to tear the delicate skin of the medial portion of the ear canal skin. The tympanomastoid suture line and the tympanosquamous suture line are visualized. The surgeon then utilizes a No. 6400 Beaver blade to make the superior and inferior incisions of the vascular strip, and a No. 7200 Beaver blade is used to make a parallel to annulus cut ~4 to 5 mm lateral to the annular rim (**Fig. 2.7**). The vascular strip is then held anteriorly in the self-retaining retractor. This exposure now allows the surgeon to visualize the pathology of the tympanic membrane more clearly.

Now with the 20-gauge suction in the surgeon's left hand and a small round dissector in the right hand, the cuff of medial ear canal skin is elevated to the annulus. Generally a relaxing incision is made on the medial ear canal wall skin of the tympanic bone, 4 to 5 mm lateral and parallel to the inferior annulus. The middle ear is entered by elevating the cuff of skin until the fibrous annulus is visualized inferior to

the chorda tympani nerve, and then elevating the annulus inferiorly and anteriorly. At this point, the middle ear may be well visualized (**Fig. 2.8**).

Control of Disease

These initial steps are performed in all cases. Once the middle ear is well exposed, the decision for which type of tympanoplasty technique is determined (underlay, overlay, or over–under). The indications for over–under tympanoplasty technique are outlined in **Table 2.2**.

Middle ear cholesteatoma, granulation tissue, and diseased mucosa are dealt with at this time. If a mastoidectomy is required to remove tissue safely from the middle ear or if there is disease in the mastoid then an intact canal mastoidectomy with facial recess approach is employed. Further treatment decisions are made as described in other chapters of this book.

Preparation of Tympanic Membrane Remnant

When the disease process is under control, the tympanic membrane remnant is prepared for grafting. A rim of tissue is removed from the perforation edge to remove diseased tissue or mucosal thickening and encourage migration of healthy epithelium and the mucosal layer. Now for those patients where an over–under tympanoplasty is to be employed, the malleus is clearly visualized by elevating the tympanic membrane. The periosteum of the malleus is incised with a fine

Table 2.2   Indications for Over–Under Tympanoplasty

Perforations or retractions that abut the malleus
Large or near-total perforations
Severe malleus retraction
Significant anterior tympanosclerosis
Anterior middle ear cholesteatoma
Ossicular reconstruction

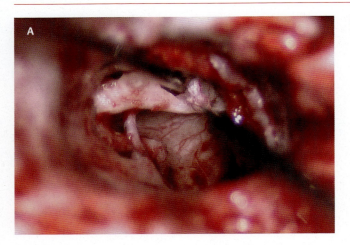

Fig. 2.9 (**A,B**) Incising the periosteum of the malleus.

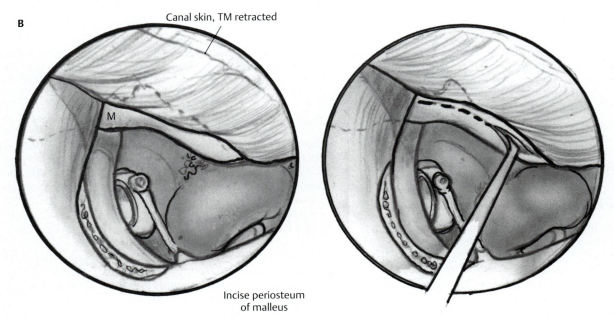

Canal skin, TM retracted

Incise periosteum
of malleus

sharp needle (**Fig. 2.9A,B**). This periosteal cuff is then used to elevate the tympanic membrane off the short process of the malleus, the neck of the malleus, and the long process of the malleus to the fibrous umbo area (**Fig. 2.10**). At this point either a microalligator-type scissors or the laser is used to remove the remnant from the malleus (**Fig. 2.11**).

Internal Packing

When there is significant middle ear mucosal disease or severely retracted malleus, a fitted piece of silicone sheeting (Silastic, Dow Corning, Midland, MI) is placed on the entire promontory area (0.25 mm thickness). Generally the sheeting is fashioned to ~10 to 12 mm in diameter with a small cutout where the stapes is located. Gelfoam (Pharmacia, Peapack, NJ) is cut into 8 mm discs, saline soaked, and dried on a Silastic cutting block. One or two discs are used to pack the eustachian tube. Another disc is placed on the Silastic sheet medial to the malleus. If more is necessary to fill the

middle ear cleft an 8 mm disc cut in half is used to fill the space.

Placement of Graft

The parchment-like fascia graft is now removed from the Teflon block and trimmed to the appropriate size. Generally, for near total perforations, the fascia is trimmed to a tongue shape with the anterior edge ~10 mm in diameter. The graft is then made ~15 mm in length. This allows the graft to be tucked under the anterior, inferior, and superior bony annulus, over the malleus, and then onto the posterior bony canal wall (**Fig. 2.12**). The remnant of tympanic membrane is then placed onto the lateral surface of the graft, and the remainder of the ear canal skin flaps is replaced into the normal position (**Fig. 2.13**). A disc of EpiFilm (bioactive lamina composed of an ester of hyaluronic acid, Xomed-Medtronics, Jacksonville, FL) may be placed onto the lateral surface of the tympanic membrane, especially in large perforations. A Gel-

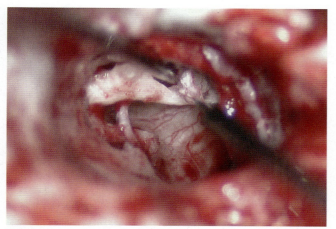

Fig. 2.10 Elevation of the tympanic membrane to the umbo and cutting from the malleus.

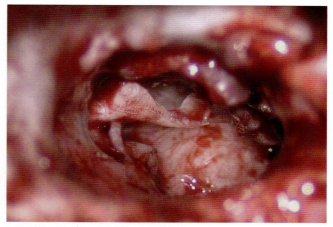

Fig. 2.11 Tympanic membrane off the malleus.

foam 8 mm disc is placed lateral to the EpiFilm (or primarily) and then antibiotic ointment applied through a 14-gauge soft catheter on a 5 mL syringe is placed onto the Gelfoam, filling the anterior sulcus of the ear canal.

The self-retaining retractors are removed, hemostasis is secured, and the T incision is closed with an absorbable suture. The postauricular incision is sutured with an absorbable suture in a subcuticular manner. No skin sutures are necessary.

The ear canal is then visualized under the operating microscope and evacuated of blood, making sure not to suction onto the graft, but placing the vascular strip skin onto the fascia graft. This is held into position with a nonabsorbable sponge moistened with an antibiotic steroid suspension. A mastoid dressing is placed.

Postoperative Care

The mastoid dressing is removed the first postoperative day. The ear canal sponge is moistened with the antibiotic steroid suspension a couple of times each day. The pack is removed on the first postoperative appointment in about a week.

◆ Cartilage Tympanoplasty

The cartilage graft has been utilized in certain tympanoplasties for over 40 years. Situations that may benefit from the use of cartilage with or without perichondrium are for scutum defects, for repair of posterior retraction pockets, or for total tympanoplasties, for the recurrent retracted middle ear cleft, and for recurrent perforations after previous failed tympanoplasties. Although similarly used as fascia for reconstruction, the rigid quality of cartilage tends to resist resorption and retraction. The anticipation of conductive hearing loss when using cartilage to reconstruct the tympanic membrane is of concern, but most reports state that there is not a statistically significant difference in advanced tympanic membrane reconstruction.[37,43] A modification of Dornhoffer's

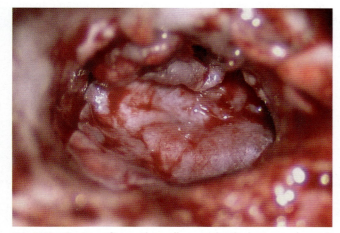

Fig. 2.12 Fascia graft over the malleus, under the bony annulus and onto posterior boney canal wall.

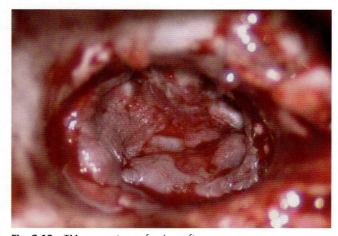

Fig. 2.13 TM remnant over fascia graft.

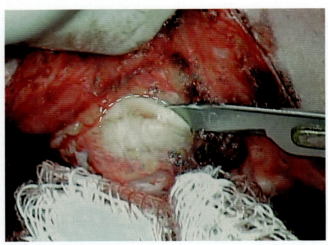

Fig. 2.14 Harvesting cartilage and perichondrium from the cimbum concha. With the surgeon's finger in the cimbum, the loose tissue is cleared from the plane of the perichondrium, a curvilinear incision is made through the cartilage.

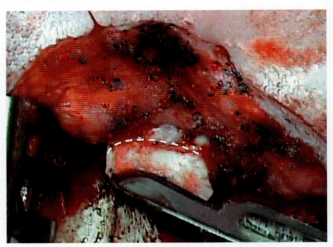

Fig. 2.15 A plane of dissection is then developed on the lateral (concave) side, leaving the perichondrium attached to the cartilage graft. The incision is then completed below (*dashed line*), and the composite graft is detached.

technique is described here. Others have used "palisade" techniques as well, in which the cartilage is scored.

The graft may be taken from the cimbum concha through the postauricular wound. The surgeon's finger placed in the cimbum can be helpful in defining its boundaries. The loose tissue over the cimbum is incised with a No. 15 blade, then the plane of the perichondrium is defined and exposed. The cartilage is then incised in a semicircular shape (**Fig. 2.14**), and the subdermal tissue is dissected away from the perichondrium on the lateral (concave) side, care being taken not to buttonhole the thin auricular skin. The incision is then completed to form a circle ~1 cm in diameter (**Fig. 2.15**), and the cartilage graft, with perichondrium on both surfaces, is removed. The graft is prepared by elevating the perichondrium away from

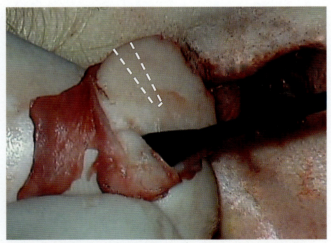

Fig. 2.16 The graft is prepared by elevating the perichondrium off the convex surface, leaving it hinged to the free edge of the cartilage. The cartilage is then trimmed to the size of the tympanic annulus, and a trough can be created to accommodate the malleus handle (*dashed lines*). This results in an island of cartilage on an oversized piece of perichondrium.

the convex surface with a duckbill elevator, leaving it hinged at one end (**Fig. 2.16**). The cartilage itself is then trimmed to the size of the tympanic membrane, and a groove can be created to accommodate the malleus handle. The final graft should be an island of cartilage on a much larger piece of perichondrium.

The tympanic membrane remnant is prepared as previously described. The cartilage graft is then used to reconstruct the entire surface area of the tympanic membrane, rotating it into position until the groove is aligned with the malleus handle (**Fig. 2.17A,B**). If the graft is of proper size, the edge of the cartilage will snap up against the posterior bony annulus and fit snugly like a manhole cover (the use of Gelfoam in the middle ear is optional with this technique). The free perichondrium is then laid against the bony canal. The tympanomeatal flap is then draped over the composite graft (**Fig. 2.18A,B**). If the perforation is large, the flap can be incised at its narrowest point, usually inferiorly, and its edges advanced and rotated over the area of the perforation, to provide maximal epithelial coverage (this maneuver borrows skin from the ear canal to cover the tympanic membrane defect, which rarely poses a problem in healing).

The cartilage graft with or without perichondrium is most frequently used in the patient with a scutum defect from cholesteatoma disease (**Fig. 2.19**). It should be noted that when cartilage is used, an intact canal wall mastoidectomy has been performed either at this operation or previously. Cartilage-perichondrial grafts are also selectively used in canal wall down procedures. We advise the use of perichondrium attached to the cartilage as the graft of choice. The cartilage is then trimmed from the perichondrium as needed to repair the particular defect.

The tragus is an alternative place for harvesting cartilage, with or without perichondrium, with over 1 cm of cartilage available. The surgeon may harvest the cartilage with perichondrium on both sides of the cartilage if tissue is needed. This series of photos is incision, identification of perichondrium, then incision through the cartilage with preservation

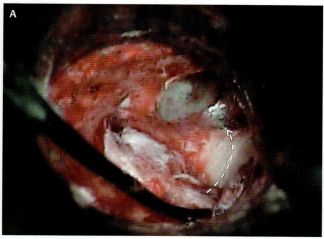

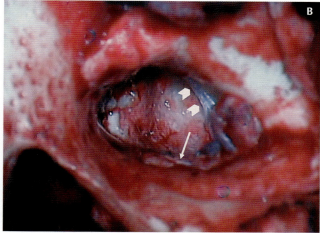

Fig. 2.17 **(A)** The cartilage graft is inserted into the ear and used to reconstruct the tympanic membrane (TM) in an underlay fashion, rotating into position until it is cinched against the bony annulus. **(B)** Cartilage graft rotated into position, with cartilage tucked under the anterior TM remnant (*arrowheads*), and the free edge of the perichondrium draped over the bony canal (*arrow*).

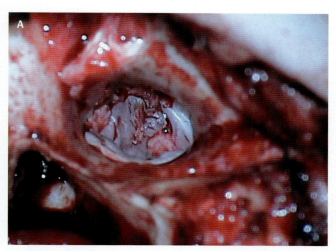

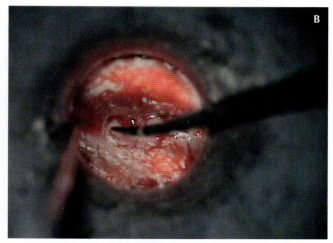

Fig. 2.18 **(A)** Tympanomeatal flap advanced and rotated over the composite graft to cover the entire tympanic membrane (TM) defect. **(B)** The tympanomeatal skin is then advanced and rotated over the TM defect to completely reepithelialize the TM.

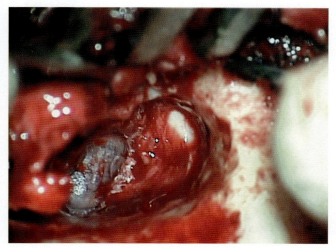

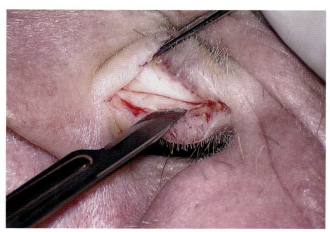

Fig. 2.19 Cartilage graft reconstruction of scutum, as well as posterosuperior tympanic membrane.

Fig. 2.20 Scissor dissection of the anterior perichondrium from the tragus cartilage.

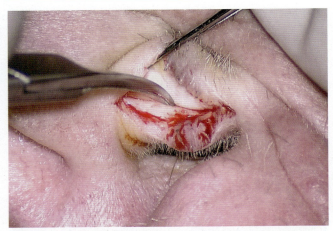

Fig. 2.21 Scissors dissection of the posterior tragal soft tissue from the tragus perichondrium and cartilage.

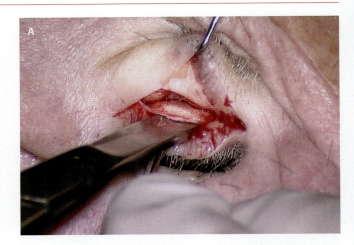

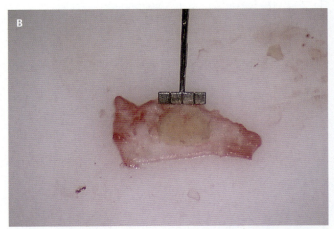

of the anterior perichondrium in its anatomical position (**Figs. 2.20, 2.21,** and **2.23**). Removal of cartilage from the perichondrium is then accomplished, with the necessary size determined by the pathology. The perichondrium is then draped over the malleus with the cartilage to fit the defect of the tympanic membrane and scutum if necessary, then the remaining perichondrium is laid onto the posterior bony canal wall (**Figs. 2.23** and **2.24**).

◆ Laser-Assisted Myringoplasty

Laser-assisted myringoplasty is a minimally invasive surgical technique for a select group of patients, using the CO_2 laser to reduce or eliminate tympanic membrane atelectasis. Our study revealed a significant reduction in the redundant tympanic membrane. Tympanic membrane atelectasis is the loss of normal contour and elasticity of the tympanic membrane as a result of persistent negative middle ear pressure.

Fig. 2.22 Trimmed cartilage block attached to the perichondrial tissue.

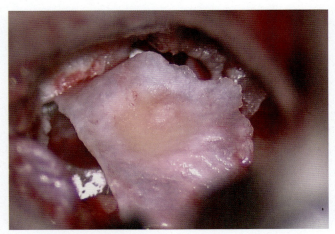

Fig. 2.23 Perichondrial cartilage graft in place to repair the scutum and the tympanic membrane defect.

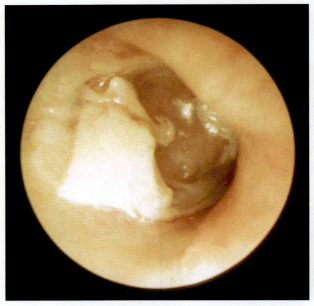

Fig. 2.24 Perichondrial cartilage graft in place to repair the scutum and the tympanic membrane defect.

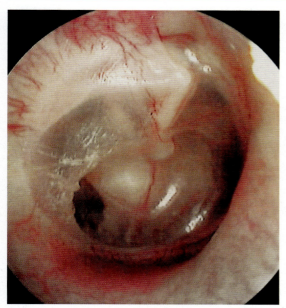

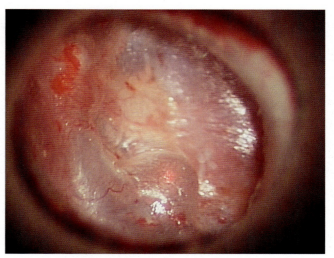

Fig. 2.26 **(A)** Posterior atelectactic tympanic membrane previously onto promontory and incus and stapes, inflated with general anesthesia.

Fig. 2.25 Atelectatic tympanic membrane with a small retraction pocket.

Atelectasis occurs in advanced chronic otitis media with or without effusion and often with chronic otorrhea. Atelectasis predisposes the patient to adhesive otitis, tympanic membrane atrophy, cholesteatoma formation, ossicular erosion, hearing loss, dizziness, and perforation. Atelectasis is one of the most difficult problems encountered with the tympanic membrane due to its chronicity and progression of severity over time. If identified in the early stages of retraction, atelectasis can be halted or even reversed by placing ventilation tubes to eliminate negative pressure in the middle ear. We have observed that even after placement of middle ear ventilation tubes to alleviate the effect of eustachian tube dysfunction, the tympanic membrane will often remain atelectic or "floppy," with persistence of a retraction pocket (**Fig. 2.25**).

The redundancy and weakening of the tympanic membrane must be addressed. Traditionally, the approach is formal tympanoplasty with resection of the atelectatic portion of the membrane and reconstruction with a fascia graft. We sought to develop a minimally invasive clinical technique in which a CO_2 laser is used to cause a thermal contraction of the tympanic membrane. This allows for tissue tightening and reduction in size of the atelectatic pocket without tympanoplasty. The laser can also be used to lyse fibrous scar bands arising on the perimeter of the atelectatic region of the tympanic membrane. Lysis of the fibrous bands also promotes reduction in the size of the atelectatic region of the membrane (**Figs. 2.26, 2.27,** and **2.28**).

Our conclusion has been consistent, reproducible descriptions of tympanic membrane atelectasis are necessary.

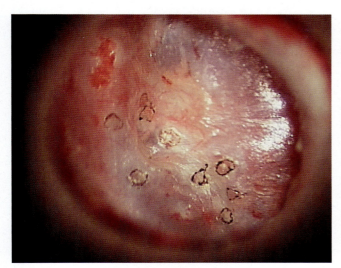

Fig. 2.27 Laser contracted tympanic membrane.

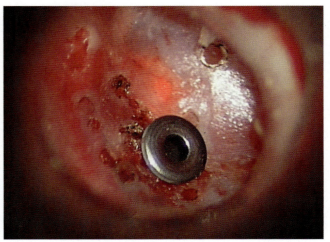

Fig. 2.28 Laser contracted tympanic membrane (TM) with resected herniated TM and inserted ventilation tube.

Attention must be made to size, location, and depth of the atelectatic region, and this information must be conveyed in the literature via a detailed tympanic membrane atelectasis grading system. This will permit a standardized reporting format.

Laser contraction myringoplasty is a novel technique that provides the surgeon with a minimally invasive treatment option in addressing the difficult problem of tympanic membrane atelectasis. This procedure results in immediate contraction and "tightening" of the tympanic membrane tissues and avoids tympanic membrane resection or tympanoplasty in a select number of patients. Patients with persistent eustachian tube dysfunction may require ventilation tube placement. Those patients in whom a retraction pocket is present and the eustachian tube dysfunction has been resolved have the most favorable outcome.

◆ Conclusion

Over–under tympanoplasty with fascia or perichondrium and cartilage is the preferred method of tympanoplasty for the indications previously noted. Flexibility of technique is insured by the experience of the surgeon, and with any technique the surgeon should review long-term results in success of take rate, hearing improvement, and low complication rate. This technique should be included in the repertoire of the otologic surgeon.

References

1. Litton WB. Epithelial migration over tympanic membrane and external canal. Arch Otolaryngol 1963;77:254–257
2. Boxall JD, Proops DW, Michaels L. The specific locomotive activity of tympanic membrane and cholesteatoma epithelium in tissue culture. J Otolaryngol 1988;17(4):140–144
3. Mondain M, Ryan A. Epidermal growth factor and basic fibroblast growth factor are induced in guinea-pig tympanic membrane following traumatic perforation. Acta Otolaryngol 1995;115(1):50–54
4. Shimada T, Lim DJ. The fiber arrangement of the human tympanic membrane: a scanning electron microscopic observation. Ann Otol Rhinol Laryngol 1971;80(2):210–217
5. Decraemer WF, Dirckx JJ, Funnell WR. Shape and derived geometrical parameters of the adult, human tympanic membrane measured with a phase-shift moiré interferometer. Hear Res 1991;51(1):107–121
6. Hussl B, Timpl R, Lim D, Ginsel M, Wick GG. Immunohistochemical analysis of connective tissue components in tympanosclerosis. In: Lim DJ, Bluestone CD, Klein JO, Nelson JD, eds. Recent Advances in Otitis Media: Proceedings of the Fourth International Symposium. New York: BC Decker; 1988:402–406
7. Wilson JG. Nerves and nerve endings in the membrana tympani of man. Am J Anat 1911;11:101–115
8. Applebaum EL, Deutsch EC. Fluorescein angiography of the tympanic membrane. Laryngoscope 1985;95(9 Pt 1):1054–1058
9. Committee on Conservation of Hearing of the American Academy of Ophthalmology and Otolaryngology: Standard classification for surgery of chronic ear disease. Arch Otolaryngol 1964;81:204–205
10. Hippocrates. De Carnibus [in German and Greek]. Teubren BB, trans. Leipzig, Berlin, Germany; 1935
11. Banzer M. Disputatio de Audiotone Laesa. Wittenbergae: Johannis Rohrerei; 1651
12. Toynbee J. On the Use of an Artificial Membrane Tympani in Cases of Deafness Dependent Upon Perforations or Destruction of the Natural Organ. London: J Churchill & Sons; 1853
13. Blake CJ. Transactions of the first Congress of the International Otological Society. New York: D Appleton & Company; 1887
14. Berthold E. Ueber myringoplastik. Wier Med Bull 1878;1:627
15. Wullstein H. The restoration of the function of the middle ear, in chronic otitis media. Ann Otol Rhinol Laryngol 1956;65(4):1021–1041
16. Zollner F. The principles of plastic surgery of the sound-conducting apparatus. J Laryngol Otol 1955;69(10):637–652
17. Plester D. Myringoplasty methods. Arch Otolaryngol 1963;78:310–316
18. Sooy FA. A method of repairing a large marginal tympanic perforation. Ann Otol Rhinol Laryngol 1956;65(4):911–914
19. House WF, Sheehy JL. Myringoplasty: use of ear canal skin compared with other techniques. Arch Otolaryngol 1961;73:407–415
20. Plester D. Myringoplasty methods. Arch Otolaryngol 1963;78:310–316
21. Shea JJ Jr. Fenestration of the oval window. Ann Otol Rhinol Laryngol 1958;67(4):932–951
22. Austin DF, Shea JJ Jr. A new system of tympanoplasty using vein graft. Laryngoscope 1961;71:596–611
23. Tabb HG. Closure of perforations of the tympanic membrane by vein grafts: a preliminary report of twenty cases. Laryngoscope 1960;70:271–286
24. Storrs LA. Myringoplasty with the use of fascia grafts. Arch Otolaryngol 1961;74:45–49
25. Chalat NI. Tympanic membrane transplant. Harper Hosp Bull 1964;22:27–34
26. Glasscock ME III, House WF. Homograft reconstruction of the middle ear: a preliminary report. Laryngoscope 1968;78(7):1219–1225
27. Perkins R. Human homograft otologic tissue transplantation buffered formaldehyde preparation. Trans Am Acad Ophthalmol Otolaryngol 1970;74(2):278–282
28. Smith MF. Viable homograft reconstruction of the middle ear transformer mechanism and posterior osseous external canal. Trans Pac Coast Otoophthalmol Soc Annu Meet 1972;53:63–69
29. Wehrs RE. Homograft tympanic membrane in tympanoplasty. Arch Otolaryngol 1971;93(2):132–139
30. Goodman WS. Tympanoplasty: areolar tissue graft. Laryngoscope 1971;81(11):1819–1825
31. Goodhill V. Tragal perichondrium and cartilage in tympanoplasty. Arch Otolaryngol 1967;85(5):480–491
32. Patterson ME, Lockwood RW, Sheehy JL. Temporalis fascia in tympanic membrane grafting: tissue culture and animal studies. Arch Otolaryngol 1967;85(3):287–291
33. Sheehy JL, Glasscock ME III. Tympanic membrane grafting with temporalis fascia. Arch Otolaryngol 1967;86(4):391–402
34. Bojrab DI, Causse JB, Battista RA, Vincent R, Gratacap B, Vandeventer G. Ossiculoplasty with composite prostheses: overview and analysis. Otolaryngol Clin North Am 1994;27(4):759–776
35. McFeely WJ Jr, Bojrab DI, Kartush JM. Tympanic membrane perforation repair using AlloDerm. Otolaryngol Head Neck Surg 2000;123(1 Pt 1):17–21
36. Jackson CG, Glasscock ME III, Nissen AJ, Schwaber MK, Bojrab DI. Open mastoid procedures: contemporary indications and surgical technique. Laryngoscope 1985;95(9 Pt 1):1037–1043
37. Dornhoffer J. Cartilage tympanoplasty: indications, techniques, and outcomes in a 1,000-patient series. Laryngoscope 2003;113(11):1844–1856
38. Austin DF. Transcanal tympanoplasty. Otolaryngol Clin North Am 1972;5(1):127–143
39. Glasscock ME III. Tympanic membrane grafting with fascia: overlay vs. undersurface technique. Laryngoscope 1973;83(5):754–770
40. Wehrs RE. Grafting techniques. Otolaryngol Clin North Am 1999;32(3):443–455
41. Hough JV. Tympanoplasty with the interior fascial graft technique and ossicular reconstruction. Laryngoscope 1970;80(9):1385–1413
42. Kartush JM, Michaelides EM, Becvarovski Z, LaRouere MJ. Over-under tympanoplasty. Laryngoscope 2002;112(5):802–807
43. Gerber MJ, Mason JC, Lambert PR. Hearing results after primary cartilage tympanoplasty. Laryngoscope 2000;110(12):1994–1999

3

Ossicular Chain Reconstruction

Success in ossicular chain reconstruction (OCR) is achieved when a mobile tympanic membrane and a secure sound-conducting mechanism to the inner ear fluids are present in the absence of infection or cholesteatoma. Early thoughts on hearing restoration following surgery for chronic ear disease date to some of the work of Wullstein and Zollner.[1,2] This chapter reviews the mechanics of hearing, the history of OCR, the materials used for OCR, and factors predicting success in OCR.

◆ Acoustic Mechanics

The normal human middle ear couples sound from the low-impedance sound energy in the ear canal through the tympanic membrane and ossicles to the relatively high impedance of fluid within the cochlea. In the absence of this mechanism, ~97% of the sound waves reaching the oval window would be reflected or lost due to the impedance mismatch between the air and cochlear fluids. The difference between these media through which sound is conducted through the external auditory canal, the ossicles, and the fluids of the cochlea makes the middle ear an impedance-matching system minimizing the energy loss. This energy loss is made up in part by the acoustic transformation theory. There is the advantage of the tympanic membrane lever, the ossicular lever, and the hydraulic lever, and the gain is ~27 to 34 dB.[3]

The *tympanic membrane lever effect* is from the tympanic membrane attachment to the malleus and provides a mechanical advantage creating amplification of energy of at least twofold gain in sound pressure at the malleus.[4] The *ossicular lever effect* consists of malleus manubrium to incus lenticular process length and provides another 1.3 sound energy gain. The *hydraulic lever effect* is the 17-fold gain from the size mismatch between the tympanic membrane and the oval window footplate area (55 mm² is the functional portion vs. 3.2 mm² for the stapes footplate).

Natural resonance and efficiency refer to the inherent anatomical and physiological properties of the external and middle ear, which allow certain frequencies to pass more easily to the inner ear.[4] The natural resonance of the external auditory canal is 3000 Hz, whereas the middle ear is 800 Hz. The tympanic membrane is most efficient in transmitting sounds between 800 Hz and 1600 Hz, whereas the ossicular chain is most efficient in transmitting sounds between 500 and 2000 Hz. These properties produce the greatest sensitivity in sound transmission between 500 and 3000 Hz, approximately those frequencies that are most important in routine conversation. Three theoretical explanations for the frequency-dependent response of the ossicular chain are presented: ossicular coupling, acoustic coupling, and stapes-cochlear input impedance. *Ossicular coupling* refers to the sound pressure gain occurring through the actions of the tympanic membrane and ossicular chain. This is important when considering results in reconstruction of the ossicular chain and tympanic membrane (types I, II, and III tympanoplasties). The maximum middle ear gain is 25 dB at 1000 Hz.

Acoustic coupling is due to the difference in sound pressures acting on the two inner ear windows. As sound energy is transmitted to the stapes footplate, fluid vibrations travel from the scala vestibuli up the cochlear partition to the helicotrema, then pass along the scala tympani toward the round window. The round window membrane is an elastic membrane that vibrates in response to sound waves traveling through the fluid medium of the inner ear. Because impulses created at the oval window must travel through the scala vestibuli and scala tympani before reaching the round window membrane, movements of the stapes footplate precede those of the round window membranes producing a phase difference between the two windows. Therefore, to transmit sound most efficiently, there must be oval window exposure and round window protection preventing sound waves from striking the round window simultaneously with the oval window and thus canceling out the vibrations. In some diseased and reconstructed ears (type IV, V tympanoplasties later described), loss of the tympanic membrane and ossicular chain can cause a hearing loss that exceeds 30 dB. This is explained by sound waves having access to both the round and oval windows causing cochlear fluid wave cancellation and interference. Shielding of the round window with cartilage or fascia results in redirection of all sound energy into the oval window.[3] Acoustic coupling theory applied allows for closure of the air–bone gap to near 20 dB. Impedance at the oval window occurs because of the annular ligament, the viscosity of the cochlear fluids, and the round window membrane. The round window impedance contribution is negligible in the normal ear. When the round window niche is occluded with fluid or fibrous tissue, the round window impedance increases, resulting in a conductive hearing loss. Sound energy is also lost overcoming the stiffness and mass of the tympanic membrane and ossicular chain.[5]

◆ History of Prostheses Development in Ossicular Chain Reconstruction

One widely accepted classification scheme breaks tympanoplasty into five subtypes. Type I tympanoplasty (myringoplasty) involves reconstruction of a tympanic membrane defect with a completely intact ossicular chain. Type II tympanoplasty involves reconstruction of an eardrum in the absence of a usable malleus; hence the tympanic membrane is brought into contact with the incus and stapes assembly. Type III tympanoplasty grafts the eardrum directly to a mobile stapes superstructure, and type IV tympanoplasty involves grafting the tympanic membrane directly to a mobile stapes footplate and shielding the round window niche from external sound. Finally, the type V tympanoplasty involves removal of a fixed stapes footplate/superstructure and replacement with a fat or vein graft combined with obstruction of the round window niche (**Fig. 3.1**).[3]

Ossicular reconstruction has been evolving with technological advances over the past 60 years. Advances of prosthesis design include biocompatible material, ease of use at the time of surgery, lighter-weight design, and means of more firm attachment to the involved structures. Prostheses now have better connection to the capitulum of the stapes, ways to attach to the malleus, and footplate shoes to help limit slippage at the footplate area.

Many materials have been used for OCR, but the ideal prosthesis should be biocompatible, capable of maintaining shape, rigid, and lightweight, with good acoustic properties. It should also be cost effective and easy to use in surgery tailored to the particular reconstructive needs of the patient. Extrusion rates for all prostheses are a factor of the material used and the recurrent diseased state of the ear. Cartilage covering all alloplastic material may help decrease the extrusion rate but is not absolutely necessary if the diseased retraction state of the middle ear has been successfully corrected with reconstruction of an aerated normalized middle ear state. Materials include polyethylene tubing, Teflon, Silastic tubing, stainless steel, titanium, gold, high-density polyethylene sponge (HDPS), bioglasses, and bioceramics.[6]

Autografts

Utilization of the patient's own incus or head of the malleus for reconstruction has always been the preferred method of reconstruction if the ossicle is present and not diseased. This is especially helpful in immediate reconstruction. The first of these materials as utilized in 1957 by Hall and Rytzner was the patient's own malleus and incus.[7] The ossicle is sculpted to the desired shape for the operative situation (stapes to malleus, footplate to malleus, stapes to tympanic membrane, or footplate to tympanic membrane) (**Figs. 3.2** and **3.3A–C**). Autologous incus grafts have been used for many years for middle ear reconstruction by modifying them to fit between the manubrium of the malleus and the stapes capitulum.[8] Autograft incus has been shown to maintain contour, shape, size, and physical integrity for at least 11 years.[3] In a series of 2200 cases, allograft and homograft prostheses yielded better hearing results than even the most biocompatible allograft prostheses.[9]

Cartilage is readily available and may be used for chain reconstruction. Autograft material, such as cartilage or bone, was one of the first materials used for ossiculoplasty.[7] Over several decades of clinical investigation into the utility of autograft prosthesis, cartilage has been shown to be an inferior implant material because it loses rigidity and mass density through neovascularization and chondritis during long-term implantation in the middle ear.[3,10] Schuknecht and Shi investigated the stability of osseous middle ear implants and found no evidence of bone erosion and little resorption.[11] Even diseased ossicles that have retained body and bulk are safe to use for reconstruction after surface stripping under the operating microscope, though if the ossicle is malformed by disease at the time of surgery, they likely have microscopic residual and should not be used in reconstruction.[12]

Homografts

To overcome some of the disadvantages of autografts, irradiated or preserved (in alcohol) homograft ossicles and cartilage were introduced in the 1960s. Homograft ossicles or cartilage are either presculpted by the processor or sculpted during surgery. Their use was common among early otologic surgeons, with hearing results and biocompatibility equivalent to autograft. The companies would preform the implant into structures of partial or total designs and in various lengths that could be used in the surgical environment. Many sizes and designs were kept in a preservative on the shelf for the surgeon to choose at the time of surgery. The environment surrounding homograft material has changed since 1986 with wider awareness of risk toward communicable diseases (human immunodeficiency virus, Creutzfeldt-Jakob disease).[13] Today, at least in the United States, the use of homografts for ossicular reconstruction has drastically fallen.

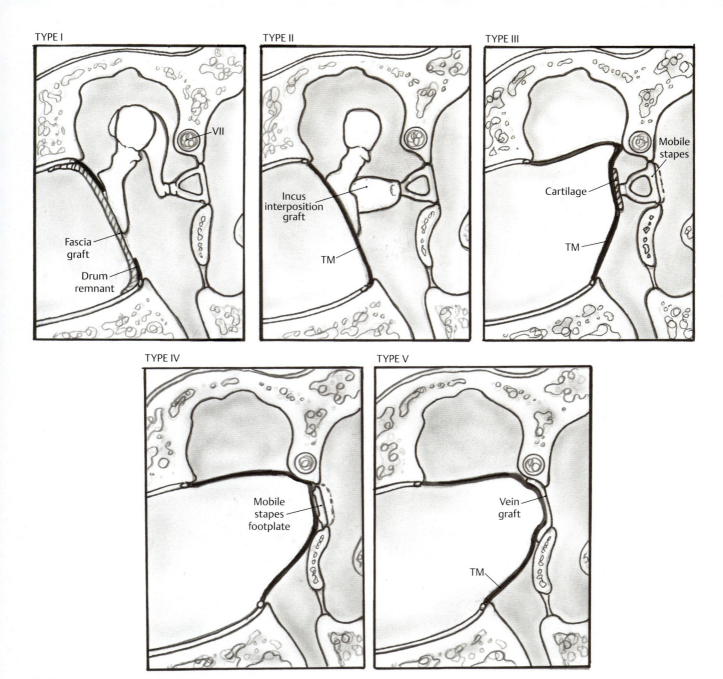

Fig. 3.1 I–V type of tympanoplasties.

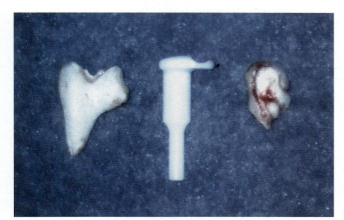

Fig. 3.2 Incus and malleus head before shaping.

Alloplasts

Initially there were prostheses designed of polyethylene, then Teflon, and finally porous polyethylene. Many of the early materials demonstrated high rates of migration, extrusion, and reactive fibrosis. Finally HDPS was developed, designed to closely mimic human bone density. HDPS is biocompatible in the middle ear, rigid, light weight, has good acoustic properties and is cost effective. If reconstruction was to go to the undersurface of the tympanic membrane, then a cartilage graft was necessary to prevent extrusion. These were made in two main designs. The *partial* prosthesis was to go from the capitulum of the stapes to the tympanic membrane with a cartilage cap, and the *total* prosthesis was to go from the stapes footplate to the undersurface of the tympanic membrane with a cartilage

A

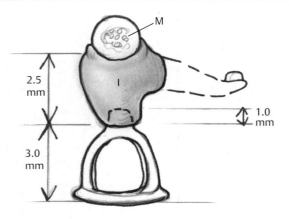

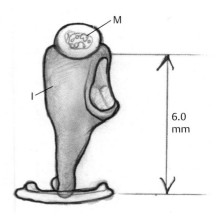

If incus too thin to drill place for 1 mm stapes capitulum head then invert incus.

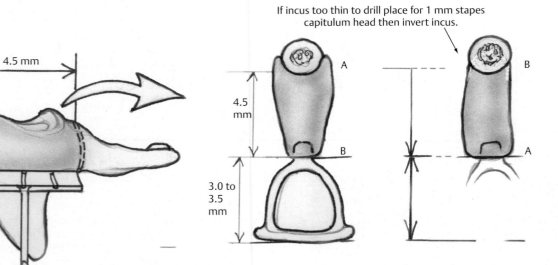

Fig. 3.3 (A) Incus shaping of different lengths as needed for surgery.

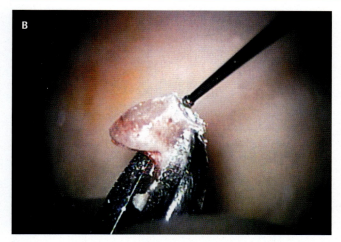

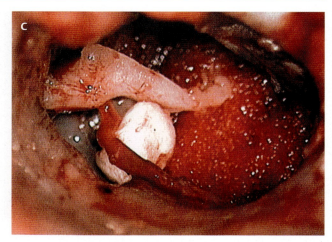

Fig. 3.3 (*Continued*) **(B)** Drilling incus with a 1 mm cutting drill and incus held in a malleus cutting forceps. **(C)** Implanted incus from the capitulum of stapes to malleus. This is an over–under tympanoplasty technique in a relatively contracted middle ear space.

cap (**Fig. 3.4**). To assist in the angulation of the tympanic membrane some porous polyethylene prostheses have been engineered to have a wire in the lumen of the prosthesis to hold the angulation of the top of the prosthesis. Extrusion rates have averaged 3 to 5% in experienced hands in a series with a 5- to 10-year follow-up.[14–16]

Hydroxyapatite (HA) is a synthetic material similar to the mineral component of bone. It is biocompatible, rigid, and has a low extrusion rate. Analysis of explanted HA demonstrates complete epithelialization and chemical bonding with osseointegration helping stability.[17,18] In most ears, placing the HA directly under the tympanic membrane is acceptable, but some authors recommend the use of a car-

tilage cap over the prosthesis when going to the tympanic membrane. This is especially true in the recurrent diseased ear. Cartilage may also provide some stability to the lateral surface, decreasing the extrusion rate.[19] Other authors state that if the middle ear condition is stable (improvement of eustachian tube function with a noncontracted middle ear space), HA may be used directly under the drum, and actually there is good integration of the implant head to the tympanic membrane (**Figs. 3.5** and **3.6**).[6] Many HA prostheses are able to connect with a groove and fit under the malleus, therefore providing lateral stability, less migration, and integration (**Fig. 3.7**). One pitfall is placement of an HA prosthesis near the scutum, which may result in unfavorable

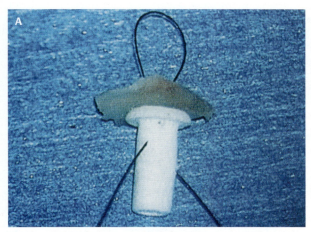

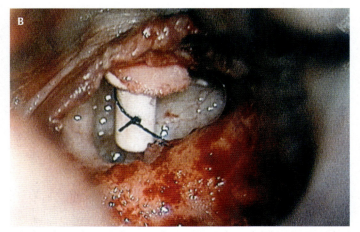

Fig. 3.4 **(A)** High-density polyethylene sponge (HDPS) partial prosthesis (PP) with cartilage graft sutured to HDPS implanted. **(B)** HDPS PP with cartilage graft sutured to HDPS placed under the tympanic membrane.

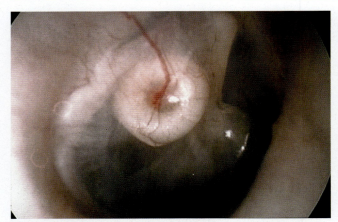

Fig. 3.5   Hydroxyapatite implant with integration and vascularity into the tympanic membrane with no malleus present.

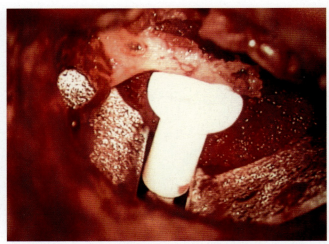

Fig. 3.6   Bojrab Universal Prosthesis cut into a partial prosthesis format, placed under the tympanic membrane in an over–under tympanoplasty surgery.

osseointegration with subsequent conductive hearing loss. Hearing results have been consistent, and extrusion rates for HA have been low (3%).[18,20]

HA is a brittle material and may fracture during operative modifications using otologic drills with diamond burrs. Because of this machining difficulty composite material of the stem of the prosthesis has been developed. HAPEX is such a design and is a combination of HA and polyethylene, and this material demonstrates the advantages in the middle ear of HA. HAPEX is more easily modified during the operation with a scalpel or diamond burr without fracturing. Although lighter in weight than HA, the HAPEX implants have some weight concerns.[5]

HA has now been made in a matrix for repairing partial ossicular necrosis. Early results have demonstrated some success in patients with incus lenticular process necrosis. This material is formatted in the operating room into a paste that is added to lengthen the incus to the capitulum of the stapes. Because most of the ossicular chain is intact and mobile, the small bridge of paste reconstitutes the connection, and excellent hearing is achieved. Long-term results are necessary to determine whether resorption will take place and recurrent surgery is necessary.

Titanium has been used for the past couple of decades for middle ear prostheses. The two most useful properties of surgical titanium are corrosion resistance and the highest strength to weight ratio of any metal. Titanium is as strong as steel but lighter in weight. Titanium is nonferromagnetic and patients may be examined with magnetic resonance imaging (MRI). The physical properties make it possible to manufacture an extremely fine with beneficial rigidity. Within the middle ear, a titanium oxide layer forms.[21,22]

Titanium middle ear implants have been made to fit most reconstructive challenges in the middle ear. When going to the tympanic membrane, a cartilage cap must be utilized. Some manufacturers have built the titanium prosthesis with an HA cap. Cartilage interface is not necessary in the middle ear that is stable with improved eustachian tube function. Some surgeons elect always to cover an HA cap with cartilage, though no controlled comparison study has been completed.

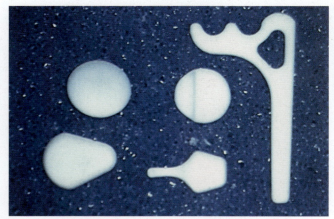

Fig. 3.7   Hydroxyapatite head variation designs with groove for malleus.

Prosthesis Design

With over 300 middle ear implants available with multiple designs, names, and materials used, we need to simplify the approach to middle ear prostheses needs and then talk about the most widely used and their benefits. Two broad categories of ossicular prosthesis should be thought of as total prosthesis (TP) and partial prosthesis (PP). The TP is designed for the middle ear situation where there is a footplate present at a

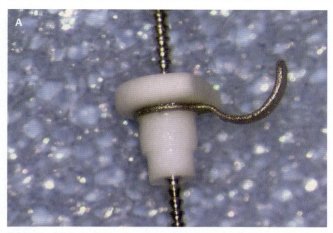

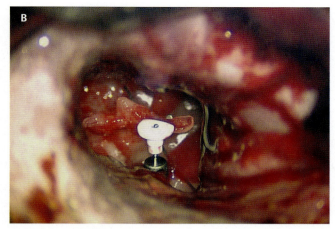

Fig. 3.8 **(A)** Bojrap Alto Prosthesis (Grace Medical). Titanium tongue extension (hook) to stabilize under the malleus. **(B)** Bojrab Alto Prosthesis Partial (Grace Medical) Under malleus in an over–under tympanoplasty.

minimum with or without a malleus. Therefore the TP prostheses may go from the footplate to the undersurface of the malleus or tympanic membrane depending on the particular situation. Rarely a tilted stapes or small, partially eroded stapes would not be suitable for a PP when the superstructure is present, and a TP may be utilized. The PP is designed for the middle ear situation where there is a stapes superstructure present with or without a malleus. Most of these will be situations where the reconstruction is from the capitulum of the stapes to the malleus or tympanic membrane. Occasionally there is an intact malleus and incus with stapes superstructure absent, and a special prosthesis may go from incus to footplate or traditional footplate to malleus.

Failure in OCR results from movement at the lateral attachment of the prosthesis, movement at the medial attachment,

extrusion of the prosthesis, or recurrent middle ear disease (poor eustachian tube function or recurrent cholesteatoma). Through prosthesis development we have worked to reduce the lateral and medial movement of prostheses. Lateral movement has been addressed by placing a groove (cradle) in the HA head (**Fig. 3.7**) or utilizing a titanium tongue (hook) to go under the malleus (**Fig. 3.8A,B**). If reconstruction is to the tympanic membrane, then some prostheses have incorporated an HA head and others with a rough-milled titanium surface to secure a cartilage cap (**Fig. 3.9**). Medially, if we are reconstructing to the capitulum of the stapes, we have made generous prostheses that simply cover the capitulum, or the capitulum and crura, essentially grabbing the stapes lightly (**Fig. 3.10A,B**). If the reconstruction is going to the footplate, we may use cartilage to stabilize the stem to the footplate, or an industry-made footplate shoe made from titanium or HDPS, to help prevent slippage (**Fig. 3.11A–E**). Lastly, to prevent mass effect, prostheses have been made lighter in weight without sacrificing rigidity, which is important for hearing results. (**Fig. 3.12A,B**).

Improvements in bioavailability, reduced footplate load, reduced operative complexity, and a greater understanding of how and when to deploy specific implants have advanced ossiculoplasty to a new era of elevated expectations. Newer prosthesis designs and materials may blend the knowledge of middle ear mechanics and biomedical engineering to create the "ideal" prosthesis.

◆ The Authors' Preferred Prostheses

Initial reconstruction utilizing homograft ossicle remains the preference for surgeons when a nondiseased incus or head of the malleus is available. If an operation is staged, the incus or the head of the malleus may be banked in the mastoid for later use. When using prosthesis for reconstruction, cost is always a factor, but this is minimized when one considers using an ossicle (either at the primary surgery or second-stage

Fig. 3.9 Cartilage onto titanium head.

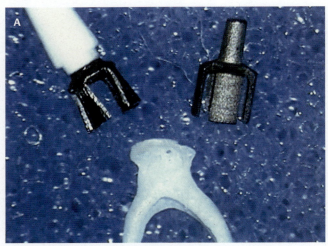
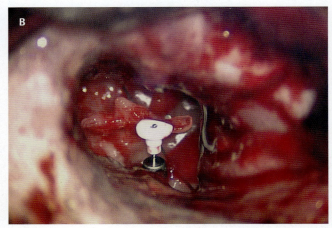

Fig. 3.10 **(A)** Titanium claw of implant. **(B)** Titanium claw onto capitulum of stapes.

approach) and the cost of operating room time and the use of an otologic drill with drill bit costs. Therefore the authors will frequently use one of the following prostheses for reconstruction either primarily or in second-stage surgery.

Titanium + HA

Multiple medical companies manufacture titanium middle ear implants with and without HA in many designs. The Grace Alto Bojrab Titanium + HA prosthesis (Grace Medical, Memphis, TN) is a lightweight, adjustable-length titanium implant available in both a total and a partial configuration with an HA head with titanium tongue extension (hook) to fit under the malleus if present (**Fig. 3.13**). The shaft length is adjusted by a provided sizing device and is shortened utilizing a simple cutting tool. This prosthesis then can be altered for another 1 mm by adjustment with the head design (**Fig. 3.14A–K**). The ability to quickly customize the length of the prosthesis intraoperatively reduces the likelihood of sizing problems seen in the purely HA prostheses that are difficult to accurately size with a diamond drill. If the malleus to stapes anatomy is unfavorable the head of the prosthesis may be covered with a cartilage cap to increase stability with the tympanic membrane and further reduce extrusion. When utilizing the total version of the Grace Alto the authors have found benefit to stabilizing the medial aspect of the prosthesis at the footplate with a titanium footplate shoe (**Figs. 3.15** and **3.16**). Similar prostheses have been made by multiple companies that have TP or PP properties. Without an HA head, a cartilage cap is always utilized. With an HA head, a cartilage cap is not utilized in the stable ear, but in conditions of continued eustachian tube dysfunction or middle ear retraction, a cartilage cap is utilized.

Universal Prosthesis

The thought of a "universal" prosthesis is desirable so that one prosthesis may be used for multiple reconstructive conditions for the patient in the operating room. In 1988, the Bojrab Universal Prosthesis was designed to be used as a TP, PP, incus sleeve, and incus to footplate prosthesis. The design has been used with HA, Hapex and HA head, Flex-HA and HA head, and HDPS and HA head, all with an HA head design with a groove to fit under the malleus if present. The Gyrus Bojrab HAPEX Universal prosthesis (Gyrus ENT, Bartlett, TN) has the benefit of composite design, with easy intraoperative modification to be utilized as a partial or total ossicular replacement prosthesis. This is particularly beneficial in trying to limit prostheses necessary to stock in the operating room. The Universal prosthesis was designed with an HA head to minimize extrusion when directly in contact with the tympanic membrane. The HA head contains a groove designed to fit under the malleus, providing stability to the lateral aspect of the prosthesis. The HAPEX (hydroxyapatite-polyethylene composite) shaft can be easily modified. HAPEX, unlike conventional HA, can be cut with a knife or drilled with a diamond drill without fracturing. The distal shaft is narrow, allowing it to function as a total prosthesis by oscillating the footplate. To utilize an intact stapes superstructure the distal shaft is trimmed, revealing a wider hollow shaft for use as a partial prosthesis, fitting over the capitulum of the stapes. In patients with

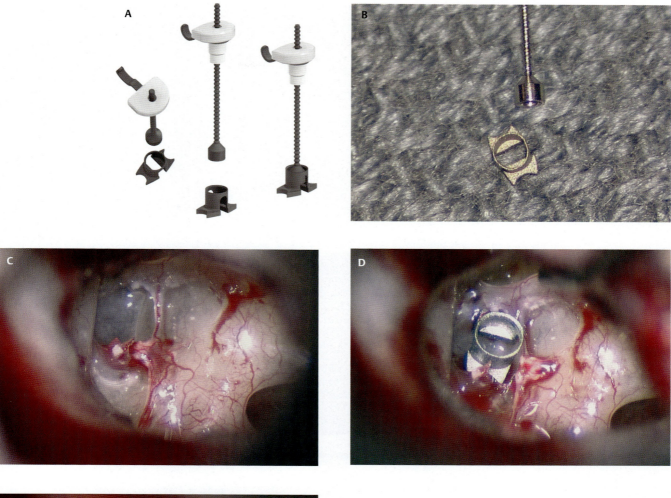

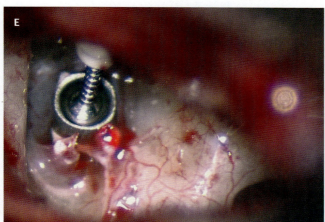

Fig. 3.11 **(A)** Titanium footplate shoe with prosthesis. **(B)** Footplate shoe and stem of Bojrab Grace Alto Total Prosthesis (Grace Medical). **(C)** Stapes footplate right ear. **(D)** Bojrab Footplate Shoe on stapes footplate. **(E)** Bojrab Grace Alto Prosthesis on Bojrab Footplate shoe on stapes footplate.

A

Prosthesis	Type	Material	Weight
Bojrab HA+Ti	Total	HA / Titanium	10 mg
Torp	Total	Dense HA	47 mg
Torp	Total	Dense HA/Flex HA	43 mg
Top	Total	Polycel	4 mg
Incus-Stapes	Total	HA / Hapex	28 mg
Incus-Stapes	Total	HA / Plasti-Pore	16 mg
Strut	Total	Dense HA	16 mg
Bojrab HA+Ti	Partial	HA / Titanium	8 mg
Porp	Partial	Dense HA	44 mg
Porp	Partial	Dense HA/Flex HA	39 mg
Pop	Partial	Polycel	6 mg
Porp	Partial	HA / Hapex	28 mg
Porp	Partial	HA / Plasti-Pore	17 mg
Strut	Partial	Dense HA	21 mg

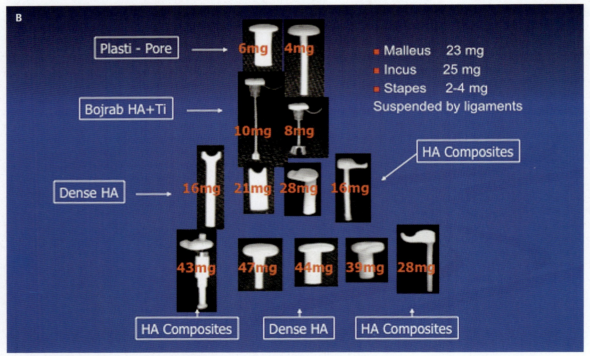

Fig. 3.12   **(A)** Prostheses weight chart. **(B)** Prosthesis pyramid of weight.

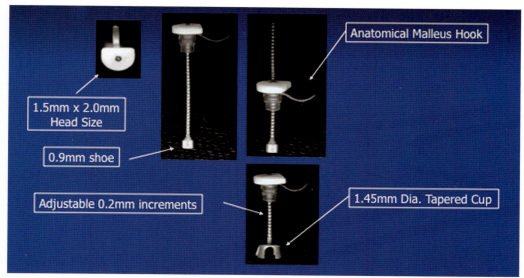

Fig. 3.13 Bojrab Grace Alto Prosthesis (Grace Medical), partial, total, and footplate designs.

an intact stapes superstructure and favorable malleus orientation, the head and distal shaft are removed, creating a hollow strut graft (**Figs. 3.17, 3.18, 3.19,** and **3.20**). From a hospital system standpoint the Universal prosthesis can be utilized in a wide variety of reconstructive situations, drastically reducing the number of prostheses needing to be stocked and reducing confusion and cost within the operative theater. Frequently a tuft of prosthesis is left on the base to provide increased integration surface for stability (**Fig. 3.21A–C**).

Hydroxyapatite Total Prosthesis and Partial Prosthesis

Multiple configurations have been made from various companies. These may be of the TP or PP configurations. Multiple sizes are available with limited surgeon adjustments possible at the time of surgery (**Fig. 3.22**). Extrusion rates are low because the prosthesis is hidden medial to the malleus, and the HA composition of the strut allows for mucosalization. As previously discussed, HA when in contact with the tympanic membrane will have the lowest extrusion rate of biomaterials presently available due to its similarity to native ossicular bone.

◆ Complications

Complications are minimized with experience of the surgeon. Frequently in second-stage surgery, an intravenous sedation technique is employed with good regional-local anesthesia using 1% lidocaine with 1/100,000 epinephrine. This prevents the problem of general anesthesia wakeup where "bucking" on the endotracheal tube may cause movement of the prostheses, even fracturing the footplate! Hearing results may be immediately obtained in the operating room theater, similar to thousands of stapes surgeries.

Immediate, intraoperative complications can occur from using an oversized prosthesis or being too aggressive in manipulating the ossicular chain. These maneuvers can result in fracture of the stapes superstructure, dislocation of the stapes or stapes footplate, tear of the annular ligament with a perilymphatic fistula, and possibly severe or total sensorineural hearing loss. Controlled microsurgical techniques and extensive practice in temporal bone laboratories and under the supervision of experienced surgeons will limit the occurrence of the foregoing. In the event of an annular ligament tear or crack in the footplate, a tissue seal of fat or fascia is recommended, combined with discontinuing the operative procedure and returning at a later date.

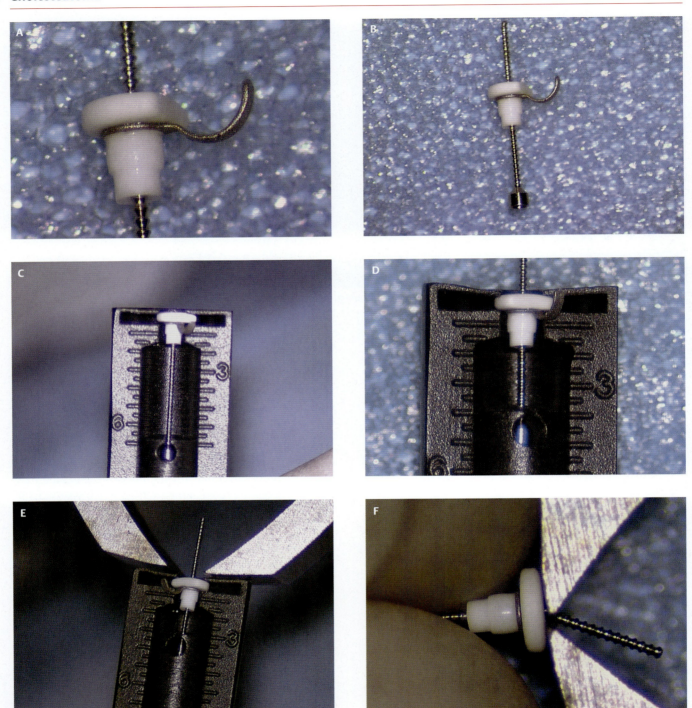

Fig. 3.14 **(A)** Prosthesis head design for total or partial prosthesis. **(B)** Bojrab Grace Alto Total Prosthesis (Grace Medical). **(C)** Bojrab Grace Alto Total Prosthesis in holder. **(D)** Bojrab Grace Alto Total Prosthesis in holder shortened. **(E)** Bojrab Grace Alto Total Prosthesis in holder cutting excess. **(F)** Bojrab Grace Alto Total Prosthesis in hand cutting excess.

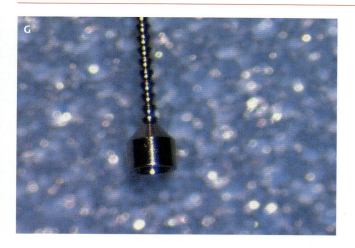

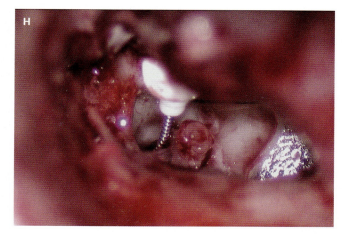

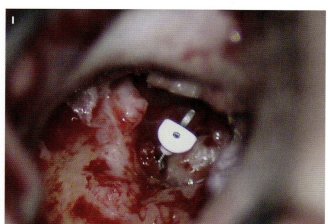

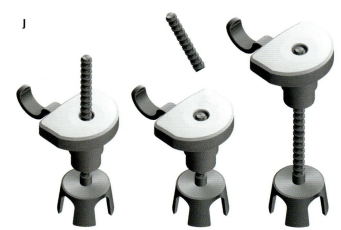

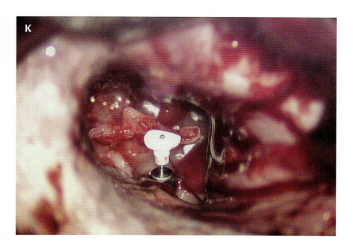

Fig. 3.14 (*Continued*)   **(G)** Bojrab Grace Alto Total Prosthesis base of stem view. **(H)** Implant in the middle ear to fit between superior to the crura of the stapes that is intact. **(I)** Implant in the middle ear to fit between superior to the crura of the stapes that is partially eroded. **(J)** Bojrab Grace Alto Prosthesis partial design. **(K)** Bojrab Grace Alto Partial Prosthesis on the capitulum of the stapes and under the malleus.

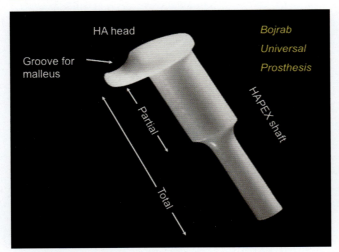

HA head

Groove for
malleus

Bojrab
Universal
Prosthesis

HAPEX shaft

Partial

Total

Fig. 3.15 Bojrab Universal Prosthesis description of utilization.

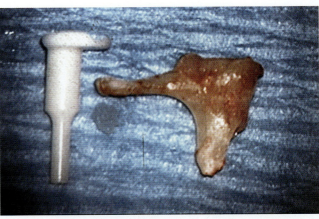

Fig. 3.16 Bojrab Universal Prosthesis with incus comparison. The prosthesis has multiple design capabilities like the potential of using an incus.

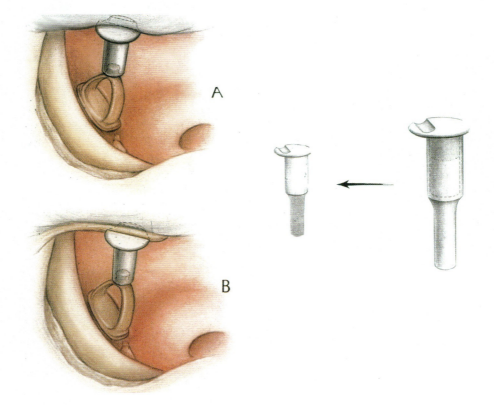

A

B

Fig. 3.17 Use of Bojrab Universal Prosthesis as partial prosthesis under the malleus or tympanic membrane.

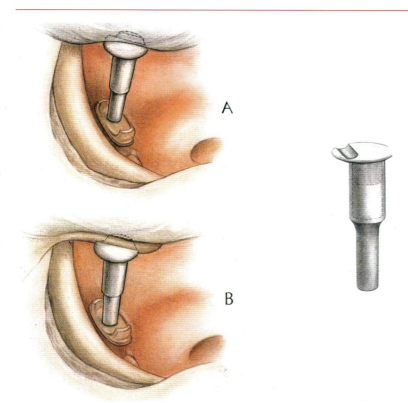

Fig. 3.18   Use of Bojrab Universal Prosthesis as total prosthesis under the malleus or tympanic membrane.

Immediate postoperative complications include vertigo and sensorineural hearing loss. Vertigo can be related to an unrecognized perilymphatic fistula or oversized prosthesis. If a complete vestibular evaluation fails to elucidate other causes middle ear exploration and revision OCR may be necessary. Sensorineural hearing loss is an uncommon com-

plication potentially related to perilymphatic fistula, serous labyrinthitis, excessive manipulation of the ossicular chain, or idiopathic causes. Treatment with corticosteroids, either oral or transtympanic, is recommended, and consideration should be given to middle ear exploration if the response is suboptimal.

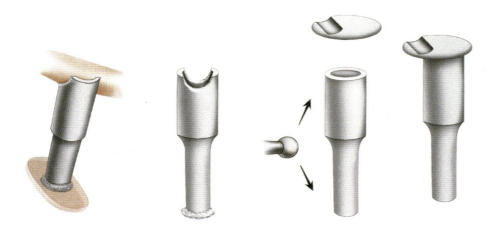

Fig. 3.19   Use of Bojrab Universal Prosthesis without HA head to go from the footplate to the malleus.

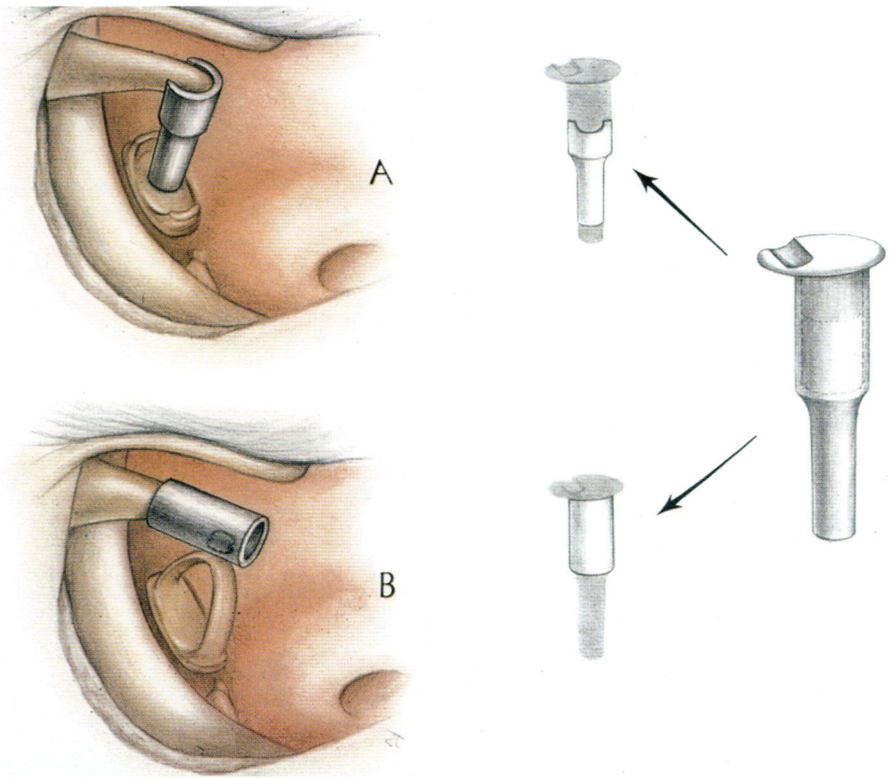

Fig. 3.20 Use of Bojrab Universal Prosthesis as incus sleeve or incus to footplate.

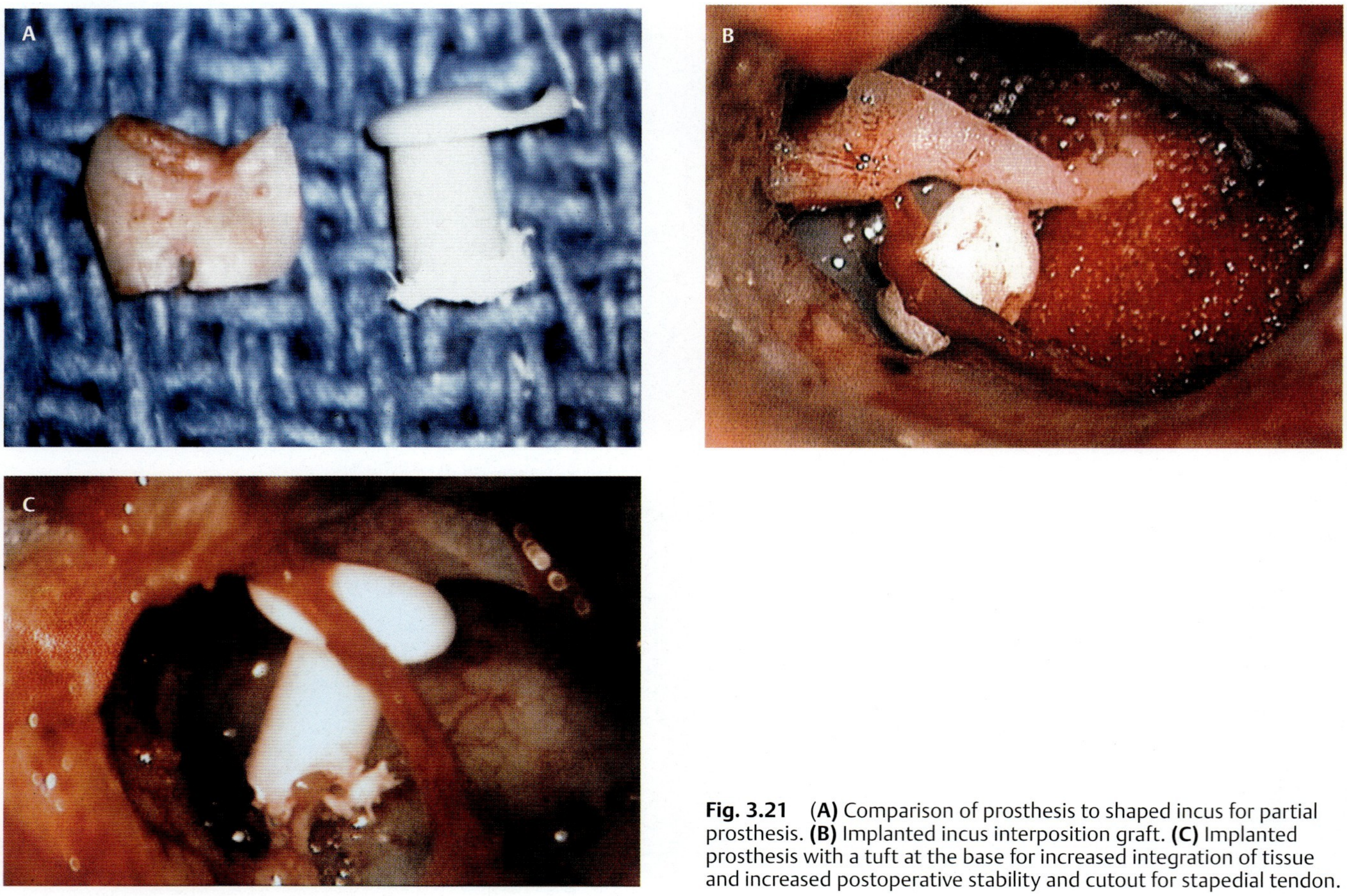

Fig. 3.21 (A) Comparison of prosthesis to shaped incus for partial prosthesis. (B) Implanted incus interposition graft. (C) Implanted prosthesis with a tuft at the base for increased integration of tissue and increased postoperative stability and cutout for stapedial tendon.

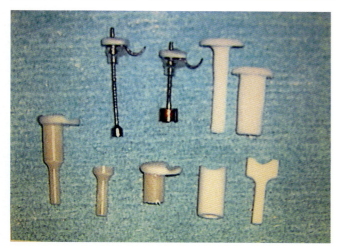

Fig. 3.22 Most used prosthesis design for total and partial reconstruction.

Delayed postoperative complications include erosion or extrusion of the prosthesis and recurrent conductive hearing loss. The cause of either may be recurrent middle ear cholesteatoma, poor healing, graft failure, dislocation of the prosthesis, ossicular fixation or erosion, or severe retraction of the tympanic membrane. In the presence of this complication the patient's candidacy for ossicular reconstruction should be reevaluated. Patients with severe eustachian tube dysfunction, extensive cholesteatoma, or persistent chronic otitis media may benefit from a type III, IV, or V tympanoplasty without the introduction of foreign material into the middle ear space.

◆ Conclusion

Ossicular chain problems are frequently encountered in otologic surgery and are amenable to reconstruction. Because various materials are used for ossiculoplasty, it is important to determine which type of prosthesis is appropriate. This decision is based on the status of the diseased ear and the surgeon's preference. Considerations must be made for the presence of absence of the malleus, the anatomical relationship of malleus to stapes, the severity of eustachian tube dysfunction, and tympanic membrane status. As newer materials are developed for use in the middle ear and implant design continues to be modified, the hearing results for patients will continue to improve.

References

1. Wullstein H. The restoration of the function of the middle ear, in chronic otitis media. Ann Otol Rhinol Laryngol 1956;65(4):1021–1041
2. Zollner F. The principles of plastic surgery of the sound-conducting apparatus. J Laryngol Otol 1955;69(10):637–652
3. Merchant SN, Ravicz ME, Puria S, et al. Analysis of middle ear mechanics and application to diseased and reconstructed ears. Am J Otol 1997;18(2):139–154
4. Goode RL, Killion M, Nakamura K, Nishihara S. New knowledge about the function of the human middle ear: development of an improved analog model. Am J Otol 1994;15(2):145–154
5. Gan RZ, Dyer RK, Wood MW, Dormer KJ. Mass loading on the ossicles and middle ear function. Ann Otol Rhinol Laryngol 2001;110(5 Pt 1):478–485
6. Hall A, Rytzner C. Stapedectomy and autotransplantation of ossicles. Acta Otolaryngol 1957;47(4):318–324
7. Hall A, Rytzner CI. Stapedectomy and autotransplantation of ossicles. Acta Otolaryngol 1957;47(4):318–324
8. Smyth G. Long term results of middle ear reconstructive surgery. J Laryngol Otol 1971;85(12):1227–1230
9. Portmann M. Results of middle ear reconstruction surgery. Ann Acad Med Singapore 1991;20(5):610–613
10. Merchant SN, Nadol JB Jr. Histopathology of ossicular implants. Otolaryngol Clin North Am 1994;27(4):813–833
11. Schuknecht HF, Shi SR. Surgical pathology of middle ear implants. Laryngoscope 1985;95(3):249–258
12. Ng SK, Yip WWL, Suen M, Abdullah VJ, van Hasselt CA. Autograft ossiculoplasty in cholesteatoma surgery: is it feasible? Laryngoscope 2003;113(5):843–847
13. Glasscock ME III, Jackson CG, Knox GW. Can acquired immunodeficiency syndrome and Creutzfeldt-Jakob disease be transmitted via otologic homografts? Arch Otolaryngol Head Neck Surg 1988;114(11):1252–1255
14. Bayazit Y, Göksu N, Beder L. Functional results of Plastipore prostheses for middle ear ossicular chain reconstruction. Laryngoscope 1999;109(5):709–711
15. Shinohara T, Gyo K, Saiki T, Yanagihara N. Ossiculoplasty using hydroxyapatite prostheses: long-term results. Clin Otolaryngol Allied Sci 2000;25(4):287–292
16. Sheehy JL. TORPs and PORPs: causes of failure—a report on 446 operations. Otolaryngol Head Neck Surg 1984;92(5):583–587
17. Hörmann K, Donath K. Is hydroxyapatite ceramic an adequate biomaterial in ossicular chain reconstruction? Am J Otol 1987;8(5):402–405
18. Grote JJ. Reconstruction of the middle ear with hydroxylapatite implants: long-term results. Ann Otol Rhinol Laryngol Suppl 1990;144:12–16
19. Meijer AG, Verheul J, Albers FW, Segenhout HM. Cartilage interposition in ossiculoplasty with hydroxylapatite prostheses: a histopathologic study in the guinea pig. Ann Otol Rhinol Laryngol 2002;111(4):364–369
20. Goldenberg RA. Hydroxylapatite ossicular replacement prostheses: results in 157 consecutive cases. Laryngoscope 1992;102(10):1091–1096
21. Dalchow CV, Grün D, Stupp HF. Reconstruction of the ossicular chain with titanium implants. Otolaryngol Head Neck Surg 2001;125(6):628–630
22. Schwager K. Titanium as a biomaterial for ossicular replacement: results after implantation in the middle ear of the rabbit. Eur Arch Otorhinolaryngol 1998;255(8):396–401

4

Mastoidectomy

◆ Anatomy of the Mastoid

The temporal bone anatomically consists of four bones: the mastoid, petrous, squamous, and tympanic (**Fig. 4.1A,B**). The pneumatized portion of the temporal bone consists of a continuous air cell tract that includes the eustachian tube, the middle ear, and the mastoid air cells (**Fig. 4.2**). From the anatomical point of view, the mastoid contains one large air cell—the *antrum*—and the periantral cells that communicate with it. Mastoidectomy, therefore, is a surgical procedure that opens the air cells of the mastoid, using a drill to remove the outer cortex and to exteriorize the contents of the temporal bone.

The mastoid has a triangular shape. The anatomical limits of the mastoid are the *tegmen* superiorly, the *posterior bony canal* anteriorly, and the *sigmoid sinus* posteriorly. The cellularity of the mastoid varies among individuals and can be well developed ("pneumatized"), diploic (marrow containing), or sclerotic (dense bone). Every mastoid, no matter how poorly developed, has a single large air cell called the *antrum* (**Fig.**

4.3). Lateral to the antrum is a thin plate of bone named the *Korner septum*. Anatomically, the Korner septum, also named the petrosquamosal septum, is an embryonic fusion plane of the squamous and petrous bones. At the base of the antrum is a dome of dense ivory bone (labyrinthine part of the otic capsule) formed by the *lateral* (or horizontal) *semicircular canal* (**Fig. 4.4**). This is the key surgical landmark in the temporal bone. The antrum communicates with the *epitympanum* (attic) superiorly, through the *aditus ad antrum*. The *fossa incudus* is the space just anterior and inferior to the aditus that houses the body of the incus. The mastoid tip is the most dependent group of air cells and is bisected by the *digastric ridge*, the indentation formed externally by the posterior belly of the digastric muscle forming the digastric groove.

The incus points to the mastoid (vertical) segment of the *facial nerve*. The facial nerve is at the same depth (lateral to medial) as the lateral semicircular canal, and is encased in a layer of dense labyrinthine bone. The mastoid segment of the facial nerve describes a shape like a candy cane, beginning just anterior to the lateral semicircular canal at the second

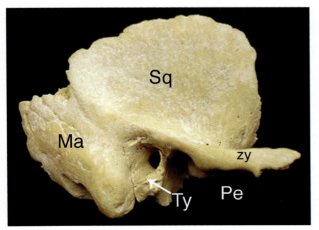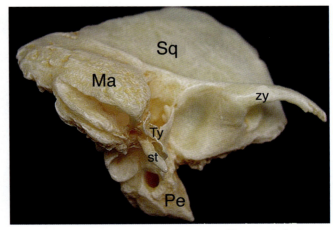

Fig. 4.1 Photographs of a left temporal bone, viewed from **(A)** laterally and **(B)** inferiorly. The four parts of the temporal bone include the squamous (Sq), tympanic (Ty), mastoid (Ma), and petrous (Pe). The zygomatic (zy) and styloid (st) process are also shown.

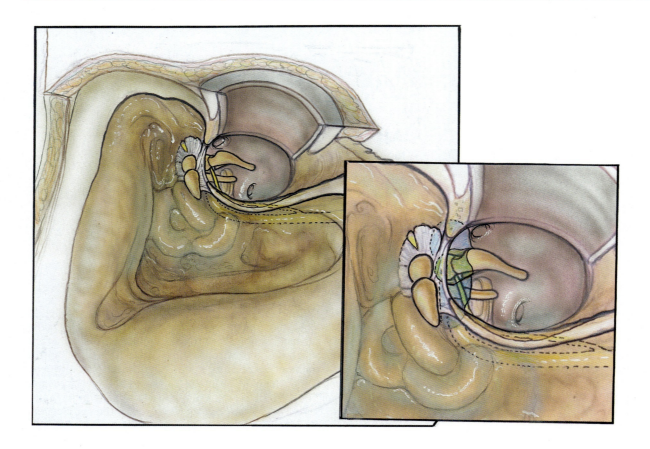

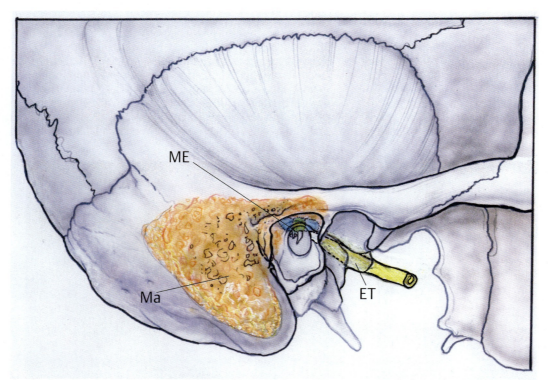

Fig. 4.2 The eustachian tube (ET), middle ear (ME), and mastoid air cell system (Ma) make up one continuous air-containing space within the temporal bone.

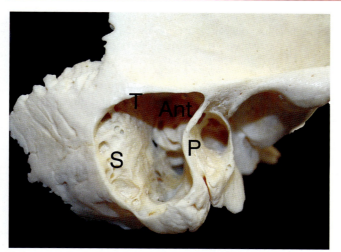

Fig. 4.3 Mastoidectomy, right temporal bone. The limits of the dissection are the tegmen (T) above, the posterior canal wall (P) anteriorly, and the sigmoid sinus (S) posteriorly. The largest air cell at the base of the mastoid cavity is the antrum (Ant).

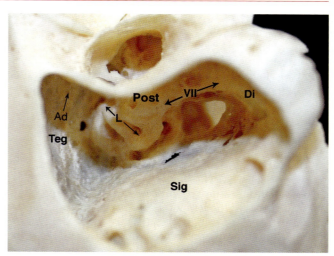

Fig. 4.4 Mastoid anatomy, as shown in a dry temporal bone dissection of the right ear and turned into a surgical position. The tegmen mastoideum (Teg), posterior bony canal wall (Post), and sigmoid sinus (Sig) form the boundaries of the surgical cavity. At the base of the mastoid antrum sits the lateral semicircular canal (L), which is an important landmark for the facial nerve (VII). The digastric ridge (Di) bisects the mastoid tip and is another landmark for the facial nerve. The aditus (Ad) is the communication from the antrum to the epitympanum.

genu and traveling inferiorly toward the mastoid tip where it exits from the stylomastoid foramen. The pneumatized cell tract just lateral to the mastoid segment of the facial nerve is called the *facial recess*. The facial recess is bounded laterally by the *chorda tympani* nerve, superiorly by the incus, and medially by the facial nerve. The facial recess can be opened surgically to create a communication between the mastoid and the middle ear. Inferiorly, the facial nerve travels close to the digastric muscle, and its sheath becomes confluent with

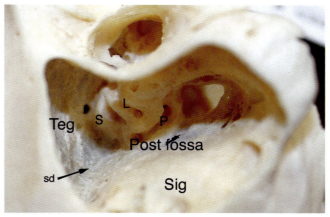

Fig. 4.5 The solid angle of bone is formed by the lateral (L), superior (S), and posterior (P) semicircular canals. The sigmoid sinus (Sig) joins the tegmen plate (Teg) at the sinodural angle (sd). The posterior fossa dural plate (Post fossa) lies anterior to the sigmoid sinus.

the periosteum of the digastric, forming a dense fibrous ring at the stylomastoid foramen.

The "solid angle" of bone in the center of the mastoid is formed by the three semicircular canals (**Fig. 4.5**). The lateral semicircular canal lies 30 degrees to the horizontal plane. The *superior semicircular canal* lies in an oblique plane and superiorly indents the tegmen to form the *arcuate eminence*. The *posterior semicircular canal* lies at right angles to the lateral semicircular canal. Medially the posterior and superior canals join to form a common crus ("crus commun").

The sigmoid sinus forms the posterior limit of the mastoid (although in a well developed mastoid a group of retrosigmoid air cells is often present). The sigmoid is so named because it describes an S-shaped course. Superiorly the sigmoid meets the tegmen mastoideum and becomes the transverse sinus. The air cells between the tegmen and the sigmoid form the sinodural angle (**Fig. 4.5**). At the depth of the sinodural angle (at the junction of the middle fossa and posterior fossa dura) is the superior petrosal sinus, which travels anteriorly to communicate with the cavernous sinus. Inferiorly, the sigmoid sinus turns in an anterior direction to enter the *jugular bulb*. The jugular bulb resides in the hypotympanum, but its location is variable, sometimes higher or lower, sometimes more anterior or posterior. The jugular bulb can be approached surgically through the retrofacial air cell tract, medial to the mastoid segment of the facial nerve.

At the depth of the mastoid, anterior to the sigmoid sinus, is the posterior fossa dura. The *endolymphatic sac* resides within the posterior fossa plate as a double fold of dura (**Fig. 4.6**). The sac is sandwiched between the posterior fossa plate and an incomplete layer of bone called the *operculum*. Superiorly, the sac forms the *endolymphatic duct*, which travels through a bony channel, the *vestibular aqueduct,* to enter the labyrinth just medial to the posterior semicircular canal.

◆ Conditions of the Mastoid

Cholesteatoma of the Mastoid

Cholesteatoma is a disease process that invades the pneumatized spaces of the temporal bone. The goals of cholesteatoma surgery are to eradicate the disease, try to restore hearing, and prevent recurrence by creating a safe, dry ear. Mastoidectomy is needed in the majority of cases to expose the disease in the temporal bone, with the exception of those that are confined to the middle ear alone.

The pattern of growth of cholesteatoma is determined by the mucosal folds described by von Troeltsch (see Chapter 1, Fig. 1.9).[1] Cholesteatomas arise from retractions of the pars flaccida in the attic or the pars tensa in the middle ear and extend upward and backward to involve the mastoid.[2] Early cholesteatomas may remain confined to the Prussak space; later on they will envelop the incus and malleus head and grow into the posterior and anterior epitympanic spaces. From there, they will extend through the aditus to fill the antrum, and eventually, all the mastoid air cells.

The procedure needed to remove a cholesteatoma is determined by the extent of the disease and the size of the mastoid. Therefore, a preoperative computed tomographic (CT) scan is often helpful to plan the operation. In cases confined to the middle ear, a tympanomeatal flap alone may provide sufficient exposure. In cases involving only the Prussak space, a limited atticotomy can be suitable. When the disease extends to the mastoid but spares the middle ear, and the disease is lateral to the head of the malleus and body of the incus, a Bondy operation might be ideal, especially if the mastoid is sclerotic. Most cholesteatomas, however, will require a mastoidectomy, and the decision to leave the canal wall up or take the canal wall down will be determined by the disease, the anatomy, the presence of complications, and the reliability of the patient, as discussed further below.

Cholesterol Granuloma

Cholesterol granuloma is a common condition that accompanies advanced cases of cholesteatoma and sometimes occurs by itself.[3] The mastoid air cells are filled with inflammatory tissue with a yellow color and a fatty consistency, and there is brown fluid with the viscosity of motor oil (**Fig. 4.7**). The middle ear may have a bloody effusion, dark blue in color, which is referred to as idiopathic hemotympanum. Histologically, there is inflammatory granulation tissue with hemosiderin, cholesterol crystals, and areas of hemorrhage. Pathologically, the condition is believed to be caused by blockage of pneumatized cells, leading to hemorrhage and later degradation of blood products. The condition is irreversible and is treated by surgical exenteration of the involved cells with reconstitution of aeration of the middle ear, epitympanum, and mastoid. A myringotomy tube alone is rarely successful in treating the condition because the tube readily becomes blocked by the thick effusion, but a tube can be a useful adjunct at the time of mastoidectomy to provide aeration and prevent recurrence of the disease.

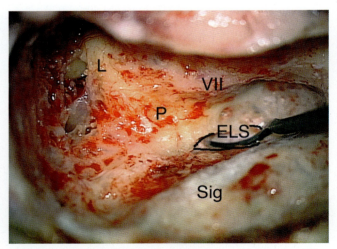

Fig. 4.6 Surgical photo of mastoidectomy, right ear. The lateral (L) and posterior (P) semicircular canals and facial nerve (VII) have been exposed. The endolymphatic sac (ELS) lies within the posterior fossa dura anterior to the sigmoid sinus (Sig).

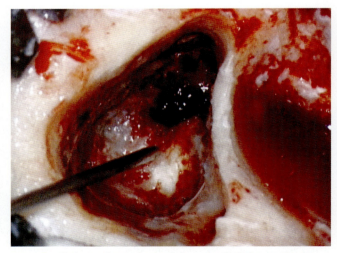

Fig. 4.7 Cholesterol granuloma of the mastoid, right ear. The air cells are filled with yellowish inflammatory tissue, and there is brown viscous fluid. The middle ear may have a bloody effusion.

◆ Surgery of the Mastoid

Classification

The terminology for mastoid surgery is not uniform. Several terms have developed to describe the different forms of mastoidectomy, summarized in **Table 4.1**. *Tympanomastoidectomy* is the general term that appears in coding manuals, but it conveys no specific information about what was done to either the middle ear or the mastoid. For the sake of clarity, it is best to describe separately the type of mastoidectomy, tympanoplasty, and ossicular reconstruction. For example, the mastoidectomy can be classified as canal wall up or canal wall down; the tympanoplasty can be classified as using a cartilage or a fascial graft; and the ossicular reconstruction can be described explicitly (eg, type III, incus interposition, etc, as covered in Chapter 3).

Canal Wall Up versus Canal Wall Down

In general, mastoidectomy can be performed in one of two ways, *canal wall up* or *canal wall down* (**Table 4.1**). The *Bondy operation* is a type of canal wall down procedure that is done in a retrograde or inside-out fashion, and which attempts to avoid the middle ear. *Atticotomy* is performed when disease is confined to the epitympanum and can be done through the mastoidectomy or through the ear canal.

The canal wall up mastoidectomy preserves the posterior bony canal wall and thereby results in normal ear canal anatomy, heals more rapidly, avoids the need for water precautions, and readily permits the use of a hearing aid. The virtue of this technique is that it avoids the problems of prolonged healing and postoperative maintenance of the mastoid bowl, but the closed cavity that results is a potential space for residual cholesteatoma to hide and for recurrent cholesteatoma to re-form. The canal wall down mastoidectomy exteriorizes the mastoid space, so that residual disease can be detected early and recurrence should (theoretically) not occur, but it carries the penalty of creating a cavity that may require periodic cleaning and water avoidance and that has the potential for drainage.

Table 4.1 Synonyms for Canal Wall Up/Canal Wall Down

Canal Wall Up (Intact Canal Wall)	Canal Wall Down
Combined approach	Atticoantrotomy, or Bondy operation
Closed technique	Open technique
Simple mastoidectomy	Modified radical (or radical) mastoidectomy

Canal Wall Up (Intact Canal Wall) Mastoidectomy

The canal wall up mastoidectomy is favored when the mastoid is very well developed, because taking the canal wall down might result in a large, troublesome cavity. When combined with a transmastoid atticotomy and facial recess opening, the canal wall up approach provides access to all areas of the mastoid and middle ear. In cases where there is no clear preference in advance for canal wall up or canal wall down, the canal wall up procedure can be performed as the initial approach and can be converted to canal wall down if the exposure proves to be limited.[4] At the time of surgery, the surgeon can accurately determine the extent of the disease and the need to take the canal wall down for more complete surgical access.

The method of canal wall up mastoidectomy is as follows. The meatus should be inspected first using a microscope and speculum. The ear canal and postauricular skin are injected with 1% lidocaine with epinephrine through a small-gauge needle to provide hemostasis and hydroplane dissection. The opening of the cholesteatoma sac in the pars flaccida or pars tensa can be inspected and bluntly probed to confirm the diagnosis and to see where the disease tracks. Tympanomeatal incisions can be created at this time, or can be performed later through the postauricular incision. A limited tympanomeatal flap can be elevated to determine the involvement of the middle ear by disease. The integrity of the incus and stapes can also be determined at this point, and the incudostapedial joint can be separated before drilling the attic (to prevent vibrational trauma to the cochlea intact ossicular chain).

A postauricular incision is made and carried down to the avascular plane lateral to the temporalis fascia, and then is continued inferiorly at the same depth, creating a flap lateral to the mastoid periosteum and sternocleidomastoid muscle (this incision transects the postauricular muscles and skeletonizes the conchal bowl from behind). Once the posterior canal skin is reached, an incision is made in the mastoid periosteum along the linea temporalis (the inferior border of the temporalis muscle) and a counterincision is made down toward the mastoid tip. The periosteum is then elevated in all directions, exposing the mastoid cortex and bony ear canal. The canal skin is then bluntly elevated from the tympanic bone. Tympanomeatal incisions can be performed through the meatus with straight and angled blades, or alternately, a U-shaped incision can be made from posteriorly, perforating the skin at a midcanal level and bringing the cuts out to 6 and 12 o'clock to fashion a conchomeatal flap (ie, a laterally based flap pedicled on the conchal skin). (Some surgeons prefer to create a "vascular strip" incision, making vertical cuts at the tympanomastoid and tympanosquamous suture lines, and a horizontal cut adjoining the two through the canal skin overlying the tympanic ring).

Once the mastoid cortex is exposed, the external landmarks are confirmed. The linea temporalis (temporal line) corresponds to the tegmen mastoideum. The cribriform area of bone just behind the tympanomeatal spine (*spine of Henle*) called the *MacEwen triangle* demarcates the position of the mastoid antrum (**Fig. 4.8**).

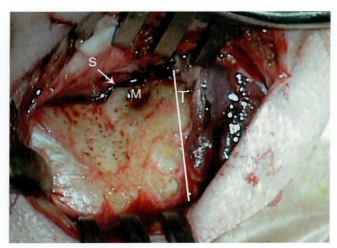

Fig. 4.8 After gaining soft tissue exposure, the external landmarks for mastoidectomy can be identified. These are the suprameatal (or Henle) spine (S), MacEwen triangle (M), and the temporal line (T, line) which is formed by the inferior border of the temporalis muscle.

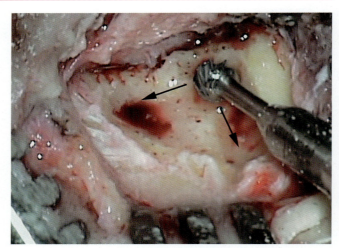

Fig. 4.9 Drilling commences parallel to the temporal line and posterior bony canal wall (*arrows*), forming a triangle with its deepest point at the MacEwen area. The MacEwen triangle is an external landmark for the mastoid antrum. The temporal line is parallel to, and never higher than, the tegmen mastoideum.

A cutting drill is used with constant suction and irrigation to create cuts in the cortical bone just inferior to the temporal line and parallel to the posterior bony meatus, with the deepest point at the MacEwen triangle (**Fig. 4.9**). A triangle of bone is removed and progressively enlarged and deepened, removing the mastoid air cells until the Korner septum is reached (**Fig. 4.10**). The internal landmarks of the mastoidectomy are the tegmen superiorly, the posterior canal wall anteriorly, and the sigmoid sinus posteriorly—these structures should be skeletonized but not violated. The Korner septum is then opened with either burr or curette to enter the mastoid antrum.

The cholesteatoma usually fills the mastoid antrum and, if the disease is extensive, it can involve the remaining pneumatized spaces of the mastoid down to the tip. Unless it is small, the cholesteatoma sac must be incised and its contents (debris) delivered before the deeper structures can be identified (**Fig. 4.11A**). The lateral semicircular canal resides at the base of the antrum; it is a dome-shaped structure formed of dense ivory bone (**Fig. 4.11B**). The lateral semicircular canal is the single most important landmark, because it "unlocks" the position of the other important structures. The lateral semicircular canal has a constant anatomical relationship to the facial nerve and stapes, and it defines the location of the facial recess opening. The mastoidectomy is then developed widely, exposing the tegmen plate superiorly and the sigmoid sinus posteriorly, and thinning the posterior bony canal wall inferiorly (**Fig. 4.11B**). All the air cells are removed down to the mastoid tip.

The attic should be opened by performing a transmastoid atticotomy (the option also exists of performing a transcanal atticotomy, described later, if the epitympanum is shallow). Generally, if the ossicular chain is intact, the incus should be disarticulated from the stapes before drilling. If extensive cholesteatoma is identified one may remove the incus at this time to further open the space and allow more exposure during the facial recess approach. The bone over the fossa incudus should be thinned to an eggshell and opened with a

curette to avoid drilling on the incus. Placing a little saline irrigation in the floor of the antrum bends the light so that the incus can be spotted early. The amount of exposure gained depends on the height of the attic (ie, the distance between the tegmen tympani and the superior aspect of the bony canal). The tegmen is followed forward toward the zygomatic root (**Fig. 4.12**). The posterior bony canal is thinned down to the level of cortical bone but not fenestrated. The bony canal is shaped like a truncated cone rather than a cylinder, so that more room is gained as one progresses medially.

Once the atticotomy is completed, the incus and malleus head will be exposed (**Fig. 4.13**). When cholesteatoma is present in the attic and antrum, the sac is incised and its contents removed with cup forceps and submitted (**Fig. 4.14A,B**). The medial wall of the sac can be maintained until it is certain that there is not a fistula of the lateral semicircular canal. If the incus body is encased in cholesteatoma it

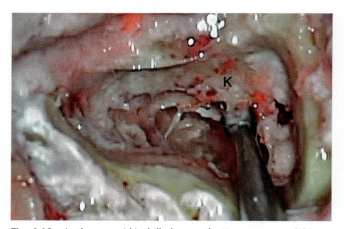

Fig. 4.10 As the mastoid is drilled open, the Korner septum (K) is often encountered. The Korner septum can be opened with a curette to avoid shredding the cholesteatoma sac with a drill.

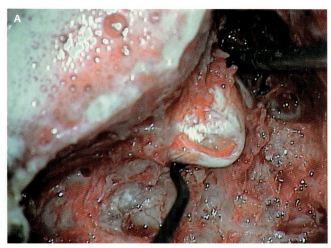
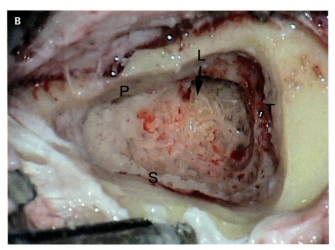

Fig. 4.11 **(A)** Cholesteatoma usually fills the mastoid antrum, and the sac must be incised and delivered before the deeper structures can be identified. **(B)** Once the antrum is opened, the lateral semicircular canal (L) can be identified in its floor, a smooth prominence of dense ivory bone. This is the key landmark to all the structures in the middle ear and mastoid. The margins of the mastoidectomy are the posterior canal wall (P), the tegmen (T), and the sigmoid sinus (S).

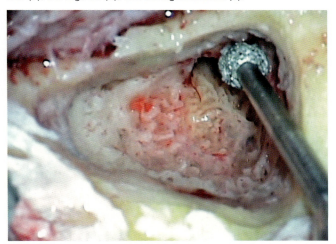

Fig. 4.12 The transmastoid atticotomy is performed by following the tegmen forward into the zygomatic root.

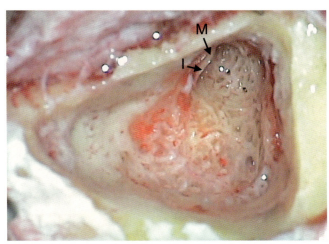

Fig. 4.13 The transmastoid atticotomy provides exposure to the body of the incus (I) and head of the malleus (M). Turning one's line of sight inferiorly would allow visualization of the tympanic segment of the facial nerve, processus cochleariformis, and bony cog, which provides access to the anterior epitympanic space.

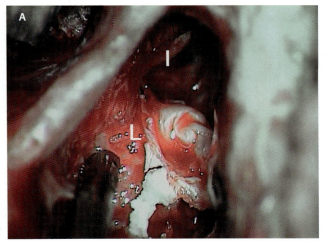
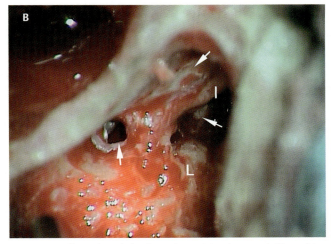

Fig. 4.14 When cholesteatoma is present in the attic and antrum, the sac is reflected and the lateral semicircular canal (L) and incus (I) are identified. **(A)** Before removal of the sac from the antrum. **(B)** After removal of the antral component; the remaining cholesteatoma matrix is seen (*arrows*) in the attic, going toward the middle ear.

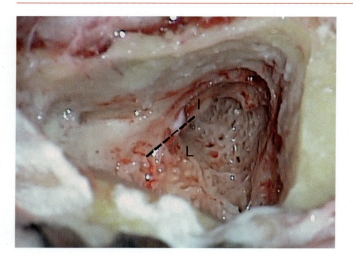

Fig. 4.15 In preparing to drill the facial recess, the facial nerve should be located, using available landmarks. The lateral semicircular canal (L) defines the medial-to-lateral depth of the facial nerve, and the incus (I) points to the facial nerve (*dashed line*). The facial recess drilling begins just lateral to the line of the facial nerve, at the level of the fossa incudus.

is removed after detaching it from the stapes (ideally performed earlier) and malleus with a curved pick. The malleus head can be detached from the manubrium with a malleus nipper. The malleus is narrowest at its neck, just above the tensor tendon; the nipper is a delicate instrument and can only be successfully closed at that point. Occasionally the sac travels lateral to the malleus and incus and the ossicles can be preserved, but this is an infrequent occurrence.

The anterior epitympanum is accessed by removing the "cog," the bony bridge found anterior to the head of the malleus that divides the epitympanic space into posterior and anterior compartments. The cog can be perforated with a small diamond burr or curette. The anterior epitympanic space is capacious, roughly equal in volume to the posterior epitympanic space, and if disease is present there the canal wall will probably have to be removed to obtain adequate exposure.

The middle ear is accessed from the mastoid through the *facial recess* approach (synonymous with "posterior tym-

panotomy"). The facial recess is a triangular space bounded by the facial nerve medially, the chorda tympani nerve laterally, and the incus buttress superiorly. The mastoid segment (vertical portion) of the facial nerve is located at the level of the lateral semicircular canal and is encased in labyrinthine (dense ivory) bone (**Fig. 4.15**). Superiorly the incus points to the facial nerve. Inferiorly the facial nerve terminates at the digastric ridge.

The facial recess is opened by drilling inferior to the fossa incudus, just lateral to the plane of the lateral semicircular canal, running the burr in parallel with the line of the facial nerve (**Fig. 4.16A,B**). The facial recess is an anatomically preformed air cell tract, gray in color and porous in texture, distinct from the ivory bone that envelops the facial nerve medially. The facial recess opening is widened in an inferosuperior direction, paralleling the facial nerve, and deepened in an anteromedial direction toward the middle ear. As drilling progresses, the burr is held at an increasingly vertical angle,

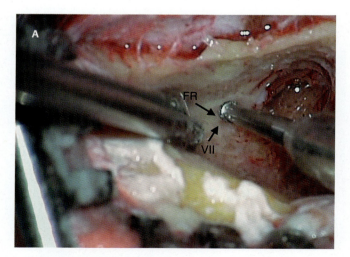

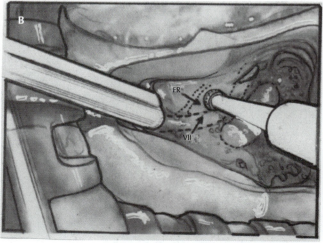

Fig. 4.16 **(A,B)** As the facial recess is opened with a diamond burr, one should note the difference in color and texture between the facial recess (FR), which is gray and porous, and the facial nerve canal (VII), which is ivory and dense. Constant irrigation should be used to ensure optimum visualization, as well as to prevent thermal trauma to the nerve.

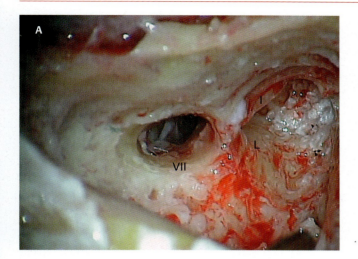

Fig. 4.17 (A,B) The completed facial recess opening allows access to the middle ear. Here, the facial nerve (VII) is skeletonized, and the relationship between the lateral semicircular canal (L), incus (I), and facial nerve is well demonstrated. Through the facial recess, the stapes, pyramidal process, and stapedius tendon can be seen. Extending the opening inferiorly would provide a good view of the round window niche.

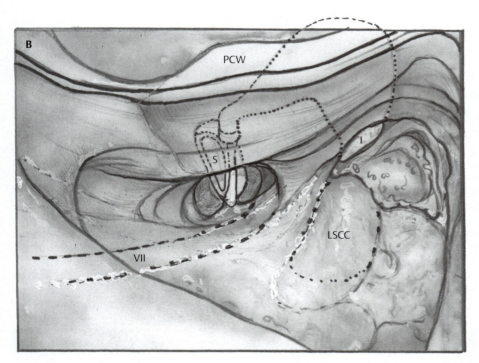

describing an arc that follows the circumference of the facial nerve. The nerve should be skeletonized but not exposed, maintaining its protective bony covering. Once the middle ear is entered, the pyramidal process and round window niche will be identified (**Fig. 4.17A,B**). The facial recess opening can be enlarged vertically by drilling the bone anterior to the facial nerve, and by drilling laterally to the tympanic annulus. It can be enlarged superiorly by removing the incus buttress. If even greater exposure is needed, the facial recess can be widened inferiorly by transecting the chorda tympani.

An adequate facial recess opening allows the surgeon to clear disease from the middle ear under direct vision (**Fig. 4.18A,B**). The problem areas of the middle ear are the region of the facial nerve second genu, the stapes superstructure, the oval window, the sinus tympani, the round window niche, the hypotympanic cells, and the protympa-

num. Opening the facial recess, removing the incus, and removing the incus buttress creates an unobstructed view into the middle ear and allows the surgeon to access all these areas (**Fig. 4.19A,B**). In some cases, the facial recess will need to be extended downward by transecting the chorda tympani nerve.

It is important to remove the mastoid air cells of the tegmen mastoideum and tegmen tympani to eliminate secreting cells in the diseased ear. The remaining mastoid cells can be exenterated, if necessary because of the extent of the cholesteatoma, by removing the bone of the sinodural angle and opening the air cells in the mastoid tip down to the digastric ridge and anterior to the sigmoid sinus down to the posterior fossa dural plate. The retrofacial air cell tract can be safely opened once the mastoid segment of the facial nerve has been skeletonized. Radical removal of all the mastoid cells

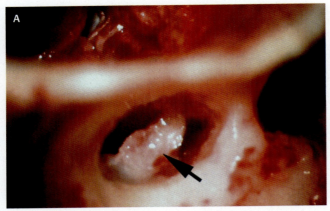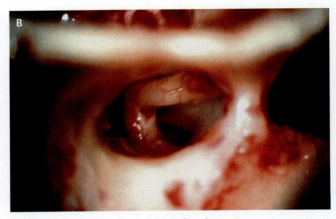

Fig. 4.18 **(A)** Facial recess approach to a cholesteatoma sac involving the left middle ear (*arrow*) before and **(B)** after dissection.

leaving only cortical bone (termed subtotal petrosectomy by Fisch)[5] is not routinely performed but is necessary in cases of extensive mucosal disease, or in cholesteatosis, where the disease is poorly encapsulated and fills all the air cells.

Surgical Decision Making: When to Take Down the Canal Wall

The decision to take the canal wall down can be made during the surgical procedure.[4] The canal wall up mastoidectomy provides access to all areas of the mastoid, epitympanum, and middle ear, and any cholesteatoma can theoretically be removed by this approach. All these regions are visible after the attic and facial recess are widely opened and the incus and malleus head and cog are removed. Dissection of the disease requires working on both sides of the canal wall, so that the patient's head will be tilted away from the surgeon during dissection of the mastoid and toward the surgeon when the surgeon is working in the middle ear. The bony canal is a barrier that can make the dissection tedious, however, and the completeness of the resection uncertain.

The primary goal of cholesteatoma surgery is the complete removal of the disease. The main disadvantage of canal wall up surgery is the chance that residual disease will remain hidden behind the intact canal wall and not be detected postoperatively. Residual disease can be left anywhere in the mastoid and middle ear cleft, but the most likely places for failure are the anterior epitympanic space, hypotympanum, and sinus tympani. More pneumatized mastoids and middle ear clefts are more dangerous because of the extension of the cholesteatoma into places that are difficult to reach. In cases with poor visualization or limited access, the canal wall will have to be removed.

The first decision point in mastoid surgery is when the attic is opened through the mastoid (transmastoid atticotomy). There must be adequate surgical exposure to completely dissect the matrix from the epitympanic spaces. As discussed earlier, the anterior epitympanic space can be quite large, and the distance between the tegmen and the bony ear canal is the limiting factor in obtaining adequate exposure. Taking down additional bone will result in an excessively large scutum defect, which can be an invitation for recurrence, even when repaired with cartilage (**Fig. 4.20A–C**). An alternative strategy in cases of anterior epitympanic cholesteatoma is to perform a transcanal atticotomy, removing the scutum widely to exte-

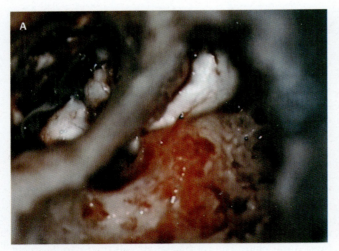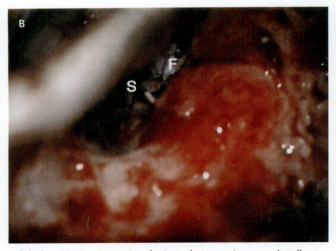

Fig. 4.19 **(A)** Facial recess approach, left ear, before and **(B)** after dissection of cholesteatoma. Removing the incus buttress, incus, and malleus head allows a clear view of the entire middle ear, including the facial nerve (F) and stapes (S). Tilting the head forward will also provide a view of the protympanum and hypotympanum through the facial recess.

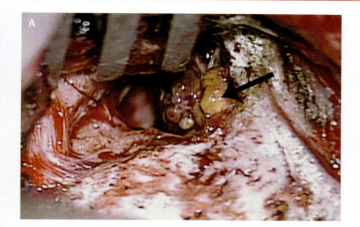

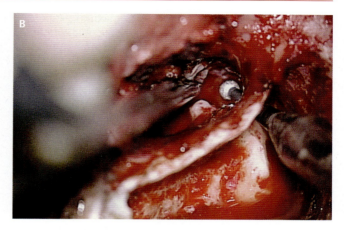

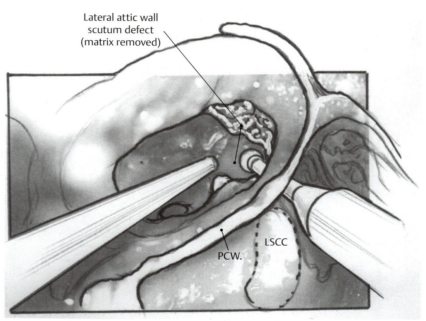

Lateral attic wall
scutum defect
(matrix removed)

LSCC

PCW.

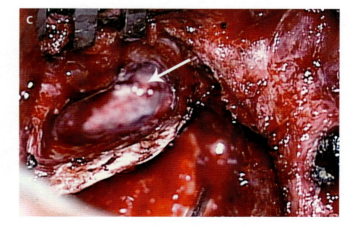

Fig. 4.20 A large scutum defect should be avoided, as it can provide a passageway for recurrent cholesteatoma to form. **(A)** An attic cholesteatoma that had eroded the scutum (*black arrow*). **(B)** A transmastoid atticotomy allows complete removal of the sac. The burr demonstrates the large scutum defect that remains. **(C)** A cartilage graft (*white arrow*) is needed to close the bony defect.

riorize the sac through the external canal. The result will be a large, shallow middle ear and the need to reconstruct the scutum with cartilage. It is often better to convert to a canal wall down mastoidectomy in these cases.

The second decision point is when the facial recess is opened to enter the middle ear. The sinus tympani is accessed through the facial recess opening, and exposure there too can be limited. Vertically widening the facial recess and removing the bone anterior to the facial nerve are ways to maximize exposure. In cases of posterior mesotympanic cholesteatoma, where the tympanic membrane is collapsed against the promontory, dissecting the sac out of the sinus tympani can be difficult, and if the sac epithelium ruptures, the likelihood of residual disease increases. Atelectasis of the posterior mesotympanum usually requires a canal wall down procedure because the posterior tympanic membrane will usually re-collapse into the middle ear space postoperatively, leading to recurrence (this is discussed further in Chapter 6, in the sections on Sinus Tympani Disease and Collapsed Middle Ear Space).

Canal Wall Down Mastoidectomy

Canal wall down mastoidectomy provides unrestricted surgical access to the middle ear and mastoid by creating an open cavity. It carries a lower rate of residual and recurrent dis-

ease than canal wall up surgery, and is generally more successful in creating a "safe" ear. However, the resultant cavity may be prone to drainage and may require periodic cleaning and "toilet" (maintenance in the office), which can be problematic, especially for children and for unreliable patients.

The canal wall down procedure is favored in certain situations: when the disease is extensive or cannot be completely removed, when the mastoid is small and sclerotic, when the patient cannot be relied upon for follow-up, when the canal wall is eroded by the disease, when the disease is recurrent, when there is a complication such as lateral semicircular canal fistula, when one is dealing with an only hearing ear.

The canal wall down procedure can be planned in advance or can be converted from canal wall up during the surgery (**Fig. 4.21A,B**). It can be performed from behind forward, or by following the disease from the attic back (inside-out or retrograde mastoidectomy). A canal wall down mastoidectomy can be performed with removal of the middle ear

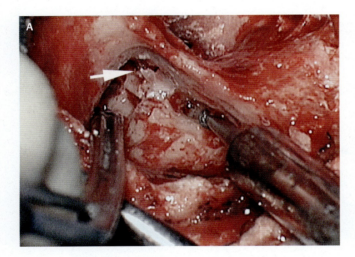

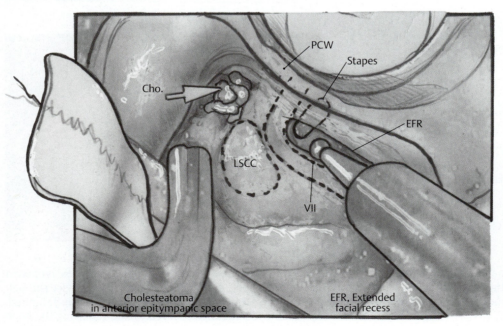

Fig. 4.21 Canal wall down mastoidectomy, right ear. **(A)** A canal wall up operation was completed first; because the disease extends to the anterior epitympanic space (*arrow*), the canal wall will be taken down. The facial recess is opened, skeletonizing the facial nerve.

contents (radical mastoidectomy), in conjunction with tympanoplasty and ossicular reconstruction, or without entering the middle ear at all (Bondy operation).

The back-to-front approach to canal wall down mastoidectomy begins with the canal wall up procedure already described. Once the mastoid landmarks are identified, the canal wall can be taken down with a cutting burr, beginning in the attic where the bony canal meets the tegmen, and progressively lowering the bone toward the mastoid segment (vertical portion) of the facial nerve. Alternatively, the facial recess can be opened first, and then the canal wall can be taken down en bloc (**Fig. 4.21A,B**). The latter approach has the following advantages: (1) the facial nerve is identified early and thus protected from surgical trauma; (2) the facial ridge is maximally lowered, resulting in a more manageable cavity; (3) the bony canal wall can be removed quickly using rongeur rather than drill; and (4) the bony canal wall can be saved and used later for cavity obliteration.

If the mastoid is well developed, it is important to exenterate all the air cells so that only cortical bone remains. Leaving pockets of cellular bone will result in postoperative mucositis and drainage. Measures that can be taken to reduce the size of the mastoid are described following here. If the mastoid is diploic, it may not be necessary to remove all the marrow-

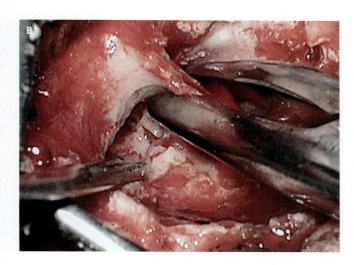

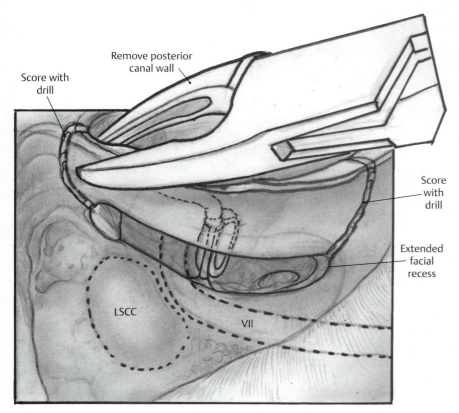

Fig. 4.21 (*Continued*) **(B)** The posterior bony canal wall can then be taken down with a rongeur.

containing spaces. Often the cavity can be sculpted into a round, well-beveled shape, using a diamond burr to polish the bleeding edges. If the mastoid is sclerotic, the disease-containing spaces can be opened, and the remaining bone can be contoured to result in a round, compact cavity without removing the entire mastoid tip.

The canal wall down mastoidectomy can also be performed in a front-to-back, or inside-out, fashion. This method is ideal when it has been decided in advance that the canal wall will be taken down, such as in a sclerotic mastoid with disease localized to the attic and antrum. This inside-out method is used when one is performing the Bondy operation, described in greater detail later in the chapter, in which a small canal wall down cavity is created without entering the middle ear. It is also used in the technique of "retrograde mastoidectomy," described by Dornhoffer,[6] in which the disease is followed from its origin in the middle ear or epitympanum, to its posterior limit in the mastoid. In Dornhoffer's method, a limited portion of the posterior canal wall is removed in the attic, and the mastoid is opened only as much as needed to expose the disease. The remainder of the canal wall is not removed, but the canal wall defect is repaired with a cartilage graft harvested from the cimbum concha to result in a closed cavity.

Creating a Manageable Cavity

Creating a manageable cavity requires four steps: (1) beveling the cavity edges; (2) lowering the facial ridge; (3) amputating the mastoid tip; and (4) creating an adequate meatoplasty.[7] Careful attention to these steps will result in a compact but well aerated cavity that can be inspected and cleaned in the office without difficulty.

The edges of the cavity are beveled while the surgeon is drilling the cortical bone near the tegmen and behind the sigmoid sinus (**Figs. 4.22A,B** and **4.23A,B**). The tegmen has a rounded contour, like the bottom of a boat, and laterally near the squamosa it turns upward. Removing the sharp ridge of bone will prevent tenting of the canal skin at this location. The position of the sigmoid sinus in the mastoid can be highly variable, and the retrosigmoid air cells can be very well developed and in some cases go all the way back to the lambdoid suture. Removing these cells can help prevent pockets that can be inaccessible in the postoperative cavity. The anterior epitympanic space is opened by removing the bony cog. The anterior canal wall bone should then be smoothed with a diamond drill, so that it becomes confluent with the anterior wall of the anterior epitympanum

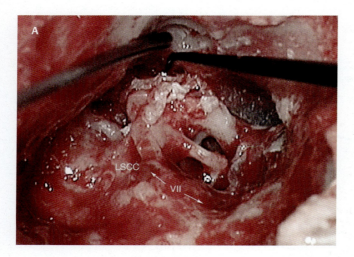

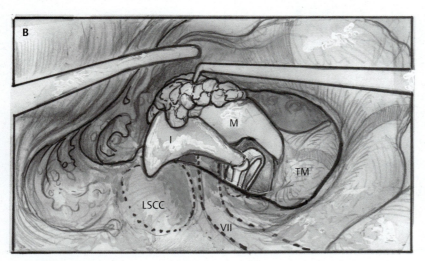

Fig. 4.22 (A,B) Once the canal wall is removed, the facial nerve is skeletonized (*arrows*), and the bone anterior to the facial nerve is thinned down with a diamond burr to provide exposure of the posterior mesotympanum. The anterior epitympanic space (instrument) has been exteriorized by removing the bony cog and smoothing out the anterior canal wall.

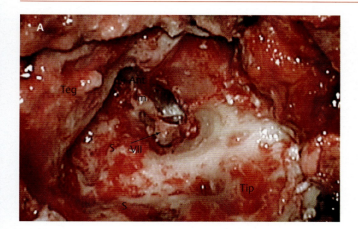

Fig. 4.23 **(A,B)** The canal wall down mastoidectomy, completed. The cortical bony edges have been beveled at the tegmen (Teg) and posterior to the sigmoid (S), and the inferior canal bone has been widened so that the base of the middle ear is confluent with the mastoid tip. (Tip). Note also that the facial ridge (VII) has been lowered and the anterior epitympanum (Ant) has been exteriorized, and all of the mastoid air cells have been exenterated.

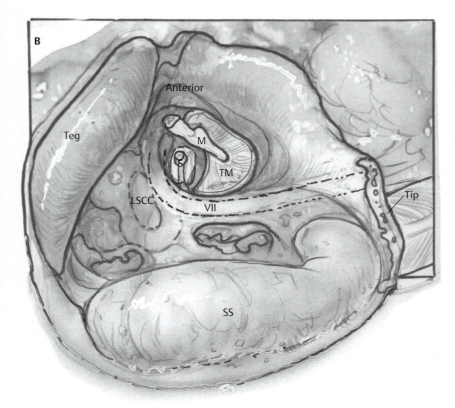

(**Fig. 4.22A,B**). Sometimes the temporomandibular joint is skeletonized during this step.

Lowering the facial ridge is essential. As already noted, opening the facial recess prior to removing the canal wall ensures that this step is performed adequately. The facial nerve should be skeletonized, leaving a thin bony covering (**Fig. 4.22A,B**). Under high magnification and using constant saline irrigation, the nerve sheath, which is white in color and has a delicate vascularity, can be identified through a thin layer of bone. When the surgical plan does not call for entering the middle ear (eg, Bondy operation), the bone anterior to the nerve can be skeletonized with a diamond burr until the fibrous annulus of the drum is seen, while preserving the cuff of distal canal skin. At the end of the procedure, this skin can be draped over the facial ridge. In surgical cases in

which the middle ear is entered, the bone anterior to the facial nerve should be removed, to gain maximal access to the sinus tympani. This is done by skeletonizing the nerve circumferentially into the middle ear space with the diamond drill and removing part of the pyramidal process if necessary. When this maneuver is completed, the round window niche, subiculum, and ponticulum should be visible.

The mastoid (vertical) segment of the facial nerve should be followed inferiorly toward the stylomastoid foramen as well, removing the triangle of bone that separates the mastoid from the hypotympanum (**Fig. 4.23A,B**). The goal is to avoid leaving a ridge of bone that prevents access to the mastoid tip cells postoperatively. The bony tympanic ring is usually quite thick, and so the bone that forms the inferior canal wall can be thinned aggressively with a coarse diamond drill.

Ideally, the floor of the ear canal can be brought down as low as the mastoid tip, avoiding a dependent group of tip cells that could later collect debris and be difficult to clean.

Amputating the mastoid tip is important to ensure that there won't be dependent cells that can drain postoperatively or harbor recurrence. In a well-developed mastoid, the mastoid tip is bisected by the digastric groove, which is formed by the posterior belly of the digastric muscle (**Fig. 4.23A,B**). A large diamond burr can be used to remove the tip cells lateral to the digastric. Once these cells are removed, the periosteum of the digastric can be exposed and be followed anteriorly where it merges with the facial nerve sheath to form a fibrous ring at the stylomastoid foramen. External to the mastoid tip, the tendinous insertion of the sternocleidomastoid muscle adheres tightly to the bone and should be stripped with a periosteal elevator. The remaining bony cortex of the tip can then be fractured with a rongeur. Once the tip is amputated, the muscles will collapse medially to obliterate this potential space. The sternocleidomastoid tendon can even be sutured to the digastric periosteum at the time of closure.

It may seem paradoxical that removing more bone will result in a smaller cavity. Beveling the cortical edges above the tegmen and behind the sigmoid, lowering the facial ridge and removing the triangle of bone between the hypotympanum and mastoid, and amputating the mastoid tip are all steps that allow the soft tissues to collapse medially, resulting in a smaller cavity (**Fig. 4.23**). Producing an adequate meatoplasty ensures that an open but compact cavity results that is easy to inspect and clean postoperatively (meatoplasty is discussed in detail in Chapter 5).

The Bondy Operation (Retrograde or Inside-Out Mastoidectomy)

The Bondy operation is an inside-out atticoantromy and is ideal for attic cholesteatoma in a compact mastoid. The principle of the Bondy operation is the exteriorization of disease to create a "safe" ear. The virtue of this operation is that it avoids the middle ear and potentially spares the hearing mechanism. Bondy first described his modified mastoid procedure in 1910,[8] at a time when otologic surgery was performed without a microscope, a drill, or antibiotic coverage, and radical mastoidectomy was the standard of care. Bondy realized that some patients with good preoperative hearing have a cholesteatoma limited to the attic exclusively, not involving the entire mastoid and middle ear. In an attempt to preserve hearing that would be destroyed in a radical mastoidectomy, he developed the more limited Bondy procedure, opening the diseased attic but leaving the eardrum and ossicular chain intact.

Characteristic and Alternative to Canal Wall Up and Down Procedures

Today's treatment for chronic otitis media with cholesteatoma has evolved from these early attempts at modification and perfection of surgical techniques and meticulous documentation of follow-up. Tympanoplasties with intact canal wall or canal wall down mastoidectomies have their indications, but modifications of these standard procedures continue to be an excellent alternative in certain subsets of patients. The distinct differences to the conventional mastoidectomies make the procedure unique.

Most important advantages of an intact canal wall are the "normal" postoperative anatomy, better hearing results, and the unrestricted lifestyle, especially for water restriction and follow-up cleaning. Especially in the pediatric population, limited mastoidectomies are favored over radical mastoidectomies due to the morbidity of leaving a mastoid cavity. But their limitation is reached when the disease process leading to a significantly contracted and sclerotic mastoid, posterior canal wall erosion, the presence of matrix over lateral canal fistula, and therefore limited mastoidectomies/atticotomies may be favorable.[9] Many authors believe that a limited atticotomy will lead to wider than normal but self-cleaning cavity,[10] an important factor in the pediatric population.

The inside-out approach described by Roth and Haeusler uses an extended Bondy technique if the cholesteatoma expands deep to the ossicles into the meso- or hypotympanum.[10] The posterior canal wall is progressively drilled inferiorly, and the middle ear space is also included into the resection, as dictated by the extent of the cholesteatoma. Instead of drilling the entire mastoid bone they recommend only removing bone overlying the cholesteatoma. This stepwise approach starts with a Bondy operation and opening the mastoidectomy leading to a radical cavity in the worst case scenario, but leaving more inferior aspects of the mastoid untouched if they are not involved with cholesteatoma.

Technique of Bondy Operation

The procedure is usually done through a postauricular incision, although a transmeatal approach using endaural incisions can be performed in a sclerotic mastoid. The object is to first exteriorize the attic by removing the scutum, then follow the tegmen tympani posteriorly until the antrum is opened as well. This is accomplished while staying out of the middle ear space.

If a postauricular approach is used, the periosteum is incised along the linea temporalis as far forward as the zygomatic root, to have exposure of the entire tegmen. The cortical bone is then removed with a cutting or coarse diamond burr until the lateral edge of the tegmen is skeletonized. The tegmen is then followed medially, and, in so doing, the scutum is progressively thinned down to an eggshell. A curette can then be used to complete the atticotomy so as to avoid drilling directly on the malleus and incus. Once this is done, the tegmen can be followed posteriorly, removing the cellular or hypocellular bone until the antrum is exposed (**Fig. 4.24**). As the drilling progresses, the mastoidectomy that is created is kept in a round shape, paralleling (and enlarging) the curve of the posterior canal wall and beveling the posterior bony edges (**Fig. 4.25**). The posterior limit of drilling is defined by the posterior extent of the antrum—it is not necessary to expose the sigmoid sinus or remove the mastoid tip. It is necessary to create a round, well-beveled cavity, so once the an-

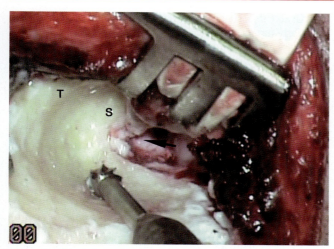

Fig. 4.24 Bondy procedure, right ear. The cholesteatoma sac grew from the posterior middle ear (*arrow*) toward the attic and antrum, and the mastoid was sclerotic. A drill is used to perform an atticoantrotomy, beginning at the tegmen (T) and thinning the scutum (S) to an eggshell, and enlarging the posterior bony canal wall to form a round, beveled cavity.

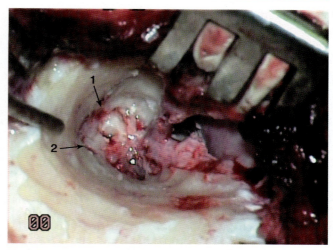

Fig. 4.25 First the tegmen is skeletonized and followed medially until the scutum is removed (1). Next, the bony opening is enlarged posteriorly, following the tegmen back to the mastoid antrum (2), and exposing the entire cholesteatoma.

trum is opened, the cortical bony edges are smoothed widely and the cavity is contoured. The posterior canal wall is removed during the Bondy procedure, beginning at the antrum and progressing inferiorly and backward (**Fig. 4.26**). The lateral semicircular canal can be used as a landmark once the antral contents are exposed and mobilized. If a diamond drill is used, the cuff of posterior canal skin that is attached to the tympanomeatal flap can be redraped over the facial ridge at the end of the procedure (**Fig. 4.27**).

Functional Results and Recurrence

DeRowe et al[11] reviewed 53 children having undergone an endaural atticotomy; even though 72% of the patients re-

quired an ossiculoplasty due to the extent of the cholesteatoma, 28% underwent a true modified Bondy mastoidectomy. Twenty-one percent of their patients needed a revision; of those, three quarters required resection of the ossicles at the first procedure. Even though the relative risk was not calculated, a trend is visible. Twenty-two percent complications were noted, of which 15% were retractions. Therefore Rakover et al stress the need for ventilation tubes at the time of surgery because they may significantly decrease the rate of recurrent cholesteatoma or the development of recurrent retractions.[12]

Bondy's findings on hearing outcome after mastoidectomy from 100 years ago were confirmed even in today's literature in a large review of more than 600 patients at the University of Berne.[10] The postoperative hearing result is largely dependent on preoperative auditory conditions. Preservation of good preoperative hearing was noted after a Bondy operation when compared with a canal wall down procedure.[13]

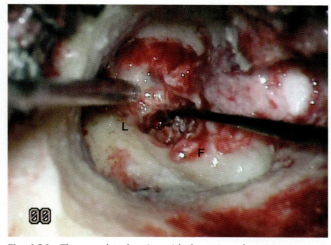

Fig. 4.26 The completed cavity, with the attic and antrum exteriorized, the facial ridge lowered down to the level of the facial nerve (F). The disease has been removed completely from the mastoid (L, lateral semicircular canal). The pick is used to raise the tympanomeatal flap to inspect the posterior middle ear.

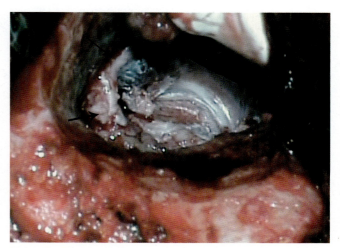

Fig. 4.27 The tympanomeatal skin is replaced (*arrows*), and used to reline the mastoid cavity.

Sanna et al reviewed their experience of 222 patients undergoing the Bondy mastoidectomy.[14] Despite a low complication rate of 19%, which include 7% residual cholesteatoma, draining cavity 7.3%, and effusion 5.2%, the long-term hearing result was excellent. Eighty-eight percent of patients had stable or even improved hearing over a 5-year period. Similar excellent hearing results were found by Berrettini et al in 53 patients reviewed with 91% hearing preservation or improvement.[15]

Today's Value of the Modified Bondy Mastoidectomy

Following Bondy's description the indication for the procedure in 1910 remains unchanged today: attic cholesteatomas or deep retraction pockets with a normal middle ear and intact ossicular chain. Sanna et al[14] summarized preoperative indications for the Bondy procedure:

- Epitympanic cholesteatoma in normal or good-hearing ear (preoperative air–bone gap, ≤25 dB) with an intact ossicular system and mesotympanum free of disease
- Epitympanic cholesteatoma in the better or only hearing ear

And intraoperative indications:

- Epitympanic cholesteatoma in the better or only hearing ear with slightly compromised but still transmitting ossicular chain

Greater awareness of ear disease and hearing problems, better health screening, and awareness of these problems among general practitioners leads to a detection of cholesteatomas at much earlier stages. But due to the progressive nature of the disease and the chance for superinfection with its potential complications, the surgical repair should be favored over observation. With the reviewed alternative technique available a mastoidectomy procedure can be tailored to the patient's needs, even if there is need for extending the Bondy mastoidectomy to an atticotomy with ossiculoplasty and tympanoplasty.

Every cholesteatoma presents in a different fashion and the otologist should be able to adapt the best procedure to maximise functional outcome in each case. As a more "minimally invasive procedure" in cases where traditionally a radical mastoidectomy might have been indicated, the Bondy mastoidectomy is an attractive alternative, not only with excellent hearing results but also as an easy and quick approach.

Atticotomy

The attic consists of three spaces, which are formed by the membranous folds described by von Troeltsch (summarized in detail and illustrated in Chapter 1). The lateral epitympanic space, or Prussak space, is bounded laterally by the scutum and medially by the head of the malleus and body of the incus. The anterior and posterior epitympanic spaces are medial to the ossicles and are separated by a bony partition familiarly named the cog.

Disease in the anterior and posterior epitympanic spaces usually requires removal of the incus and head of the malleus, and almost always involves a mastoidectomy. However, disease confined to the Prussak space can sometimes be excised without removing the ossicles. Exteriorizing the Prussak space usually involves removing the scutum (or at least part of it), if it has not already been eroded by the disease. This procedure is a transcanal atticotomy. Alternatively, the Prussak space can be accessed through a transmastoid atticotomy.

The accompanying illustrations demonstrate the technique of transcanal atticotomy. This patient, who had recurrent otorrhea, was found to have a central tympanic membrane perforation with surrounding tympanosclerosis. A deep attic retraction pocket (or early cholesteatoma) with partial erosion of the scutum was only first discovered at surgery. Exteriorization of the attic retraction required first performing a bony canalplasty, and then removing the anterior tympanic spine with curette and diamond drill (**Fig. 4.28**). The scutum was then drilled back until the blind end of the sac could be seen and delivered forward (**Fig. 4.29**). The medial wall of the sac lifted cleanly away from the malleus and incus (**Fig. 4.30**). Mastoidectomy was not needed because it was certain that the entire sac had been removed. The scutum defect was then reconstructed with a graft of cartilage and overlying perichondrium (**Fig. 4.31**).

The reconstruction is important to prevent recurrent cholesteatoma. The problem with the transcanal atticotomy procedure is that, by removing the lateral attic wall, a potential space is created where cholesteatoma can re-form. The bony defect should be closed, and this can readily be done with a composite graft of cartilage and perichondrium. The cartilage–perichondrial graft can be harvested through the postauricular wound from the inferior aspect of the cartilaginous ear canal, the cavum concha, or the cimbum concha,

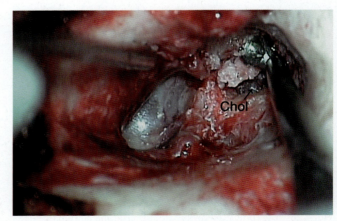

Fig. 4.28 Transcanal atticotomy, left ear. First, the bony ear canal is enlarged with a drill, then the scutum is removed with a curette to expose the attic cholesteatoma (Chol).

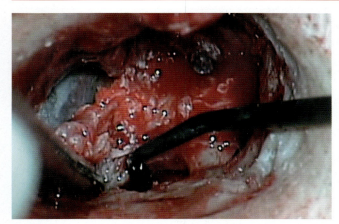

Fig. 4.29 The cholesteatoma sac is elevated off the lateral surface of the incus and malleus. The posterior and superior limits of the sac could be well seen.

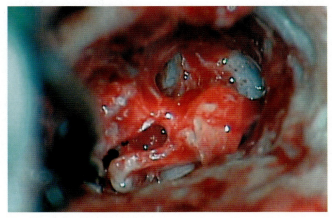

Fig. 4.30 The medial wall of the sac has been removed cleanly away from the malleus and incus.

or from the tragus through a separate incision. The perichondrium is first elevated off the convex surface of the cartilage but remains attached at the margin so that it is hinged to the perichondrium on the concave surface. The cartilage is then trimmed to the size of the bony defect, leaving it attached to the larger piece of perichondrium and wedged into place against the edges of the bony defect. The excess perichondrium can be draped over the bony canal wall, and the redundant epithelium from the sac can be used to cover it (**Fig. 4.31**).

If the attic defect is excessively large, it may be preferable to create an atticoantromy (ie, a Bondy procedure), than to attempt to close the bony defect with cartilage. This option is particularly attractive when the disease extends posteriorly to the aditus or antrum, and when the mastoid is sclerotic (this situation is demonstrated in **Figs. 4.24** and **4.25**). In such a case, a Bondy procedure will result in exteriorization of the attic (within a lower risk of recurrence) without the penalty of a large mastoid cavity (**Fig. 4.27**). It is safer to have an open canal wall down cavity than an attic defect that is not self-cleaning.

On rare occasions, nature will create its own modified radical mastoidectomy. **Figure 4.32** shows an elderly patient who had cholesteatoma but never had surgery. The disease eroded the scutum widely and effectively exteriorized itself. The result is a spontaneous atticotomy, a self-cleaning attic defect that does not become infected and does not collect squamous debris. This is a safe ear that may occasionally require cleaning in the office but will not require surgery.

Another way of managing disease in the attic is through a transmastoid atticotomy. This method is desirable in situations where a relatively large attic cholesteatoma develops behind a relatively small scutum defect, as illustrated in **Fig. 4.33A**. In this technique, a canal wall up mastoidectomy is performed, and the attic is opened from behind, by drilling forward from the mastoid into the zygomatic root cells. This requires identifying and skeletonizing the tegmen mastoideum and following it forward toward the middle ear, and by thinning (but not perforating) the posterior bony canal wall. Recall that the bony canal tapers from lateral to

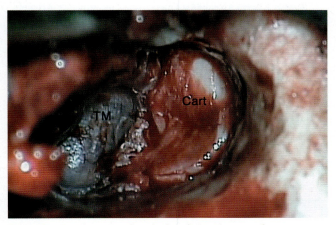

Fig. 4.31 Cartilage–perichondrial graft (Cart) repair of scutum defect. TM, tympanic membrane.

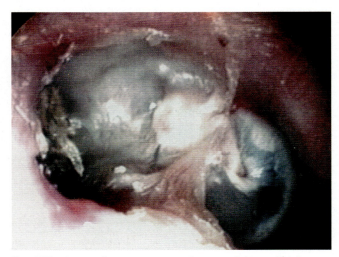

Fig. 4.32 A case of a spontaneous atticotomy, right ear. This is a cholesteatoma that eroded the scutum widely, creating an auto-mastoidectomy that is exteriorized and self-cleaning. This patient required no surgery.

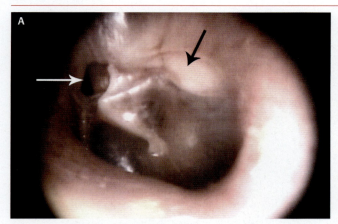
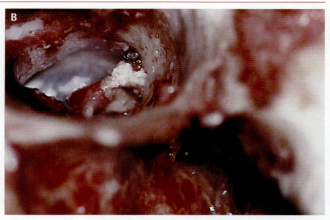

Fig. 4.33 **(A)** An attic cholesteatoma in which a relatively large sac (*black arrow*) developed behind a relatively small scutum defect (*white arrow*). **(B)** After the transmastoid atticotomy is completed, the sac can be completely freed from the incus and delivered toward the middle ear.

medial, so that it has the shape of a truncated cone rather than a cylinder. The disease can then be delivered toward the middle ear and removed (**Fig. 4.33B**). The small scutum defect that remains can be closed with a cartilage graft. If the disease is confined to the Prussak space and an intact ossicular chain can be preserved, a normal-appearing ear with normal hearing can be expected. The advantage of this approach is that the bony scutum is maintained (at least as much of it as had not been eroded by the disease), and protects against recurrence by forming a rigid barrier (bone is more reliable than cartilage in this respect). The disadvantage is that it is less direct than the transmeatal approach to the attic, and that the surgical exposure is limited by the distance between the tegmen and the bony canal wall. The vertical height of the attic varies from one individual to the next, and may sometimes be quite narrow. In an average temporal bone, the volume of the attic is roughly equal to the volume of the middle ear, and it should be possible to view the entire incus body and malleus head through the transmastoid approach. If the incus and malleus head are removed, it should also be possible to gain access to the anterior epitympanic space by removing the bony partition or cog. A diamond drill should be used for a transmastoid atticotomy, and the microscope should be tilted upward to view the tegmen during drilling. Care should be taken not to violate the tegmen (which could lead to encephalocele) or injure the dura (cerebrospinal fluid leak), as well as not to perforate the posterior bony canal (creating a potential channel for cholesteatoma to re-form from external canal skin).

References

1. Proctor B. The development of the middle ear spaces and their surgical significance. J Laryngol Otol 1964;78:631–648
2. Jackler RK. The surgical anatomy of cholesteatoma. Otolaryngol Clin North Am 1989;22(5):883–896
3. Miura M, Sando I, Orita Y, Hirsch BE. Histopathologic study of the temporal bones and eustachian tubes of children with cholesterol granuloma. Ann Otol Rhinol Laryngol 2002;111(7 Pt 1):609–615
4. Parisier SC. Management of cholesteatoma. Otolaryngol Clin North Am 1989;22(5):927–940
5. Fisch U, Mattox D. Micro-surgery of the Skull Base. New York: Thieme; 1988
6. Dornhoffer JL. Retrograde mastoidectomy with canal wall reconstruction: a single-stage technique for cholesteatoma removal. Ann Otol Rhinol Laryngol 2000;109(11):1033–1039
7. Sheehy JL. Cholesteatoma surgery: canal wall down procedures. Ann Otol Rhinol Laryngol 1988;97(1):30–35
8. Bondy G. Totalaufmeisselung mit Erhaltung von Trommelfell und Gehorknochelchen. Monatsschr Ohrenheilk 1910:15–23
9. Nikolopoulos TP, Gerbesiotis P. Surgical management of cholesteatoma: the two main options and the third way—atticotomy/limited mastoidectomy. Int J Pediatr Otorhinolaryngol 2009;73(9):1222–1227
10. Roth TN, Haeusler R. Inside-out technique cholesteatoma surgery: a retrospective long-term analysis of 604 operated ears between 1992 and 2006. Otol Neurotol 2009;30(1):59–63
11. DeRowe A, Stein G, Fishman G, et al. Long-term outcome of atticotomy for cholesteatoma in children. Otol Neurotol 2005;26(3):472–475
12. Rakover Y, Keywan K, Rosen G. Comparison of the incidence of cholesteatoma surgery before and after using ventilation tubes for secretory otitis media. Int J Pediatr Otorhinolaryngol 2000;56(1):41–44
13. Shaan M, Landolfi M, Taibah A, Russo A, Szymanski M, Sanna M. Modified Bondy technique. Am J Otol 1995;16(5):695–697
14. Sanna M, Facharzt AA, Russo A, Lauda L, Pasanisi E, Bacciu A. Modified Bondy's technique: refinements of the surgical technique and long-term results. Otol Neurotol 2009;30(1):64–69
15. Berrettini S, Ravecca F, de Vito A, Forli F, Valori S, Franceschini SS. Modified Bondy radical mastoidectomy: long-term personal experience. J Laryngol Otol 2004;118(5):333–337

5

The Meatus and Cavity Management

◆ Cholesteatoma

The external auditory meatus is often not given its due importance in discussions of ear disease and ear surgery. The meatus is the point of physical entry to the ear and allows the doctor a visual portal for diagnosis of cholesteatoma and, for that matter, every form of ear pathology. Obstruction of the meatus by cerumen, disease, or foreign material causes hearing loss and discomfort, and these are often the first symptoms that alert the patient to a problem. Surgical management of the meatus has great importance in controlling the functional outcome after otologic surgery because the meatus allows for proper surveillance in the postoperative period, and for detecting and managing recurrent disease. Primary cholesteatoma of the external canal and a related condition, keratosis obturans, also merit special discussion.

◆ Anatomy and Considerations

The external auditory canal (EAC) is unique in that it is lined by keratinizing squamous epithelium, which does not penetrate the skin surface anywhere else in the body. This fact is what makes cholesteatoma possible. Embryologically, the EAC derives from the first branchial cleft, an invagination from the external surface of the face, which meets the derivative of the first pharyngeal pouch, the middle ear cleft, at the plane of the tympanic membrane (the tympanic membrane is formed by an outer ectodermal layer, a middle fibrous mesodermal layer, and an inner mucosal endodermal layer, as reviewed in Chapter 2) (**Fig. 5.1**).

The anatomy of the external meatus is not complex. The EAC is formed of bone in its medial two thirds and cartilage in its lateral one third. The bony portion is formed mainly by the *tympanic bone*. The tympanic ring is horseshoe shaped and is deficient superiorly in the area called the *notch of Rivinus*. The anterosuperior end of the tympanic bone forms the tympanosquamous suture, and the posterosuperior end forms the tympanomastoid suture (**Fig. 5.2**).

The cartilaginous ear canal forms the meatus itself. The bony–cartilaginous junction is the narrowest part of the EAC and the point at which cerumen often becomes trapped. The cartilage that forms the external meatus is contiguous with the auricular cartilage. Anterosuperiorly, the cartilage is deficient at the *incisura*, the area between the root of the helix and the *tragus*. Inferiorly the cartilage can be quite thick. The tragal–antitragal notch is at the 6 o'clock position of the meatus (**Fig. 5.3**).

The skin that covers the cartilaginous ear canal is relatively thick and contains specialized apocrine glands that produce cerumen. The skin that covers the tympanic bone is very

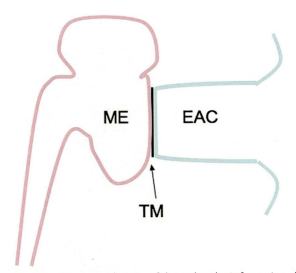

Fig. 5.1 Schematic drawing of the embryologic formation of the ear: the middle ear (ME) is formed from the first pharyngeal pouch, and the external canal is formed from the first pharyngeal cleft. The tympanic membrane (TM) is formed at the plane where these structures meet, and consists of three layers—endoderm (pink), mesoderm (black), and ectoderm (light blue).

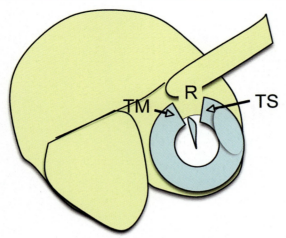

Fig. 5.2 Schematic drawing of a right temporal bone, showing the tympanic bone (*light blue*) forming the bony external auditory canal. The bone is horseshoe shaped, with a deficiency superiorly, the notch of Rivinus (R), and communicating anteriorly at the tympanosquamous (TS) and posteriorly at the tympanomastoid (TM) sutures.

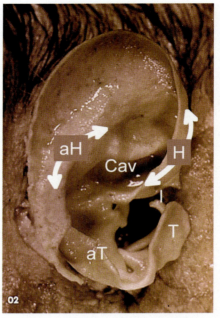

Fig. 5.3 Cadaver dissection of auricular and external auditory canal cartilage, right ear. T, tragus; aT, antitragus; I, incisura; H, helix; aH, antihelix; Cav, cavum concha. (Courtesy of Dr. Simon Parisier.)

thin, not hair bearing or glandular, and very sensitive to pain or pressure. The skin that covers the notch of Rivinus superiorly, between the two suture lines, is looser, and is referred to as the *vascular strip* because it has its own blood supply (**Fig. 5.4A,B**). The tight ear canal skin is contiguous with the epithelial lining of the pars tensa of the tympanic membrane. The vascular strip skin is contiguous with the pars flaccida and the skin overlying the manubrium up to the umbo. A hydroplane injection of local anesthetic, often used to effect hemostasis at the start of ear surgery, will not cross the suture lines; therefore at least two injections are needed, one in the vascular strip and one in the inferior canal skin (injecting the four quadrants of the ear canal, as is commonly done, is superfluous).

◆ Surgical Technique of Meatoplasty

The meatoplasty is an essential step in canal wall down mastoidectomy. It is important for postoperative cavity maintenance—an adequate meatus ensures that all areas of the mastoid cavity can be inspected, and that keratin cysts or areas of inflammation can be dealt with in the office setting. The meatoplasty also ensures that the mastoid bowl is aerated, important to prevent the formation of recurrent cholesteatoma. On the other hand, an inadequate meatus may allow squamous

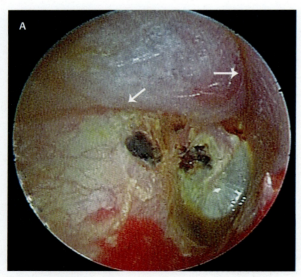

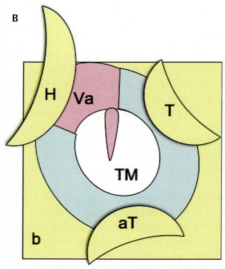

Fig. 5.4 **(A)** The vascular strip (between *arrows*) is the loose skin at the superior portion of the ear canal, between the tympanomastoid and tympanosquamous sutures (*arrows*). **(B)** The vascular strip (Va) is shown in pink, and the inferior canal skin in blue. H, root of helix; T, tragus; aT, antitragus; TM, tympanic membrane.

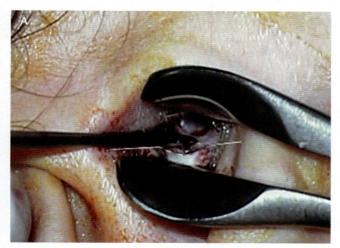

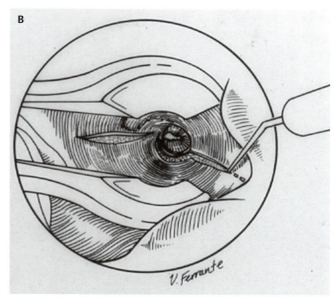

Fig. 5.5 **(A)** The meatal incisions are made through skin and cartilage, at 6 and 12 o'clock, as shown in the photo and **(B)** drawing of the right ear. The 12 o'clock incision is made in the incisura, the space between the root of the helix and the tragus. The 6 o'clock incision will be made between the tragus and antitragus.

debris to reaccumulate in the mastoid bowl, which may lead to cholesteatoma recurrence. A narrow meatus may make inspection and cleaning difficult and uncomfortable for the patient, which may discourage regular follow-up. Also, recurrent or persistent drainage may result from inadequate aeration, frequent water contamination, and insufficient hygiene.

The goal of the meatoplasty is to create a meatus that is widely patent, but not disfiguring. The overall goal of the surgery is to create a shallow, well-pneumatized cavity that is widely exteriorized to the outside. Exteriorization of the cavity is what prevents the normal skin lining from forming another cholesteatoma.

The meatoplasty is often left until the end of the surgical procedure, and if the operation is lengthy or difficult, the surgeon may try to complete this segment of the procedure hastily. However, the meatoplasty affects the surgical outcome as much as any other portion of the procedure and may be a key step in preventing cholesteatoma recurrence; thus it deserves the proper attention. Any of the steps of the meatoplasty can be performed at the start of the operation, and this may be more convenient to gain surgical exposure during the procedure.

There are many individual variations on the technique of meatoplasty, but some common elements exist.[1] *Meatal incisions* should be made through skin and cartilage and must be adequately long so as to create a *conchomeatal* (laterally based skin) *flap* that can be oriented posteriorly and into the mastoid cavity. The conchal cartilage at the meatal rim must be either *scored* or *excised*, to make the meatus larger. *Stay sutures* should be placed to ensure that the meatus remains patent. These concepts were developed by Lempert,[2] in an era when endaural approaches to the mastoid were popular.

The technique shown here incorporates those elements. The first step is to create long meatal incisions, extending laterally through skin and cartilage. A Lempert speculum can be used, with a No. 15 knife blade (or a disposable Beaver-type blade) to be sure that the full thickness is traversed (**Fig. 5.5A,B**). As this is done, the meatus can be splayed open with the leaves of the speculum. These incisions should be located superiorly at 12 o'clock, in the incisura, the skin between the root of the helix and the tragus, where there is a natural absence of cartilage; and inferiorly at 6 o'clock, between the tragus and the antitragus (these are analogous to the No. 1 and No. 2 endaural incisions described by Lempert; extending the superior incision into the preauricular sulcus can potentially allow access to the entire mastoid).

The next step is to break the spring of the conchal cartilage.[3] The cartilage that forms the meatal rim is dense—removing this allows the meatal opening to relax backward. This step is best accomplished with the surgeon's nondominant index finger in the meatal opening to serve as an anchor as well as to gauge the size of the opening. Working through the postauricular wound, the subcutaneous tissue is sharply dissected away from the conchal cartilage, staying external to the plane of the perichondrium. Once the cartilage is exposed, a crescent-shaped incision is made through the cartilage at the meatal rim (**Fig. 5.6A,B**), and this cartilage is dissected from the subcutaneous tissues and excised (**Fig. 5.7A,B**). The index finger should be easily accommodated at this point; otherwise additional cartilage can be removed with a knife or sharp scissors. The cartilage that forms the inferior meatus is often the limiting factor and should be split or excised[4] (**Fig. 5.8**). The cartilage that forms the root of the helix is also quite dense, and scoring this will often allow the meatus to be effectively enlarged. A useful measure when first learning this technique is to pass two sterile needles (25 gauge) through the conchal skin, to see where the corresponding cartilage needs to be removed.

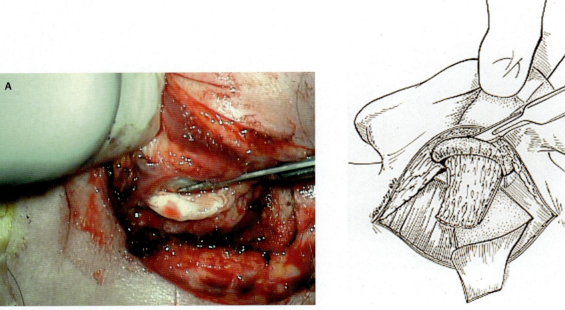

Fig. 5.6 **(A,B)** A crescent-shaped piece of cartilage is excised from posteriorly.

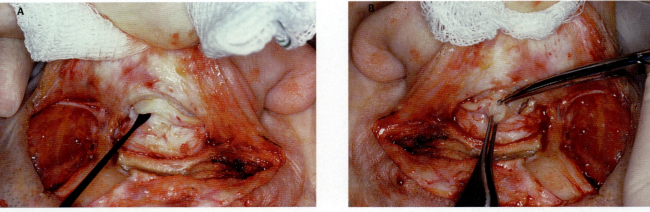

Fig. 5.7 **(A)** The cartilaginous rim of the meatus is dissected free of the subcutaneous tissue and then **(B)** excised. (Courtesy of Dr. Simon Parisier.)

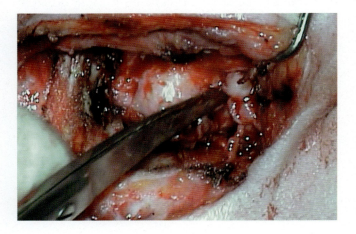

Fig. 5.8 The inferior canal cartilage is dissected.

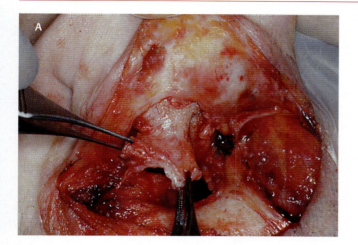

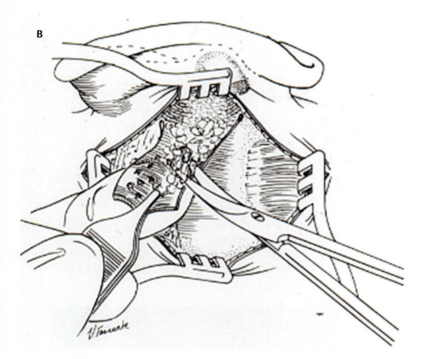

Fig. 5.9 **(A,B)** The meatal skin is thinned, to create a flap that will re-line the base of the mastoid cavity. In this example, the skin flap is thinned down to the subdermal tissue plane. (Courtesy of Dr. Simon Parisier.)

The next step is to thin the meatal skin. There are two methods that can be employed. The first excises all the fibrous subcutaneous tissue and attached cartilage to form a thin conchomeatal skin flap that can be draped over the posterior wall and floor of the mastoid cavity (**Fig. 5.9A,B**). The second method, the "musculoperiosteal flap" described by Palva (**Fig. 5.10**), leaves the fibrous tissue pedicled to the distal end of the conchomeatal flap, to provide some bulk for cavity obliteration.[5] The second method helps limit the size of the cavity but carries the risk of burying mucosal disease.

Whichever method is selected, the conchomeatal skin flap should be tacked back with stay sutures to the conchal perichondrium to create a widely patent meatal opening (**Fig. 5.11**). The flap may be directed posteriorly and somewhat superiorly toward the sinodural angle, where the cavity is largest.

Variations exist on how to make the meatal incisions. Sheehy created "vascular strip" incisions at the start of the case, pedicled superiorly, and following the tympanomastoid and tympanosquamous sutures. Others have described a bifid flap, where the conchomeatal skin is split longitudinally, with one limb directed upward and the other downward, in an effort to create a large, round meatus.[6] Z-plasties and M-plasties have also been described.[7,8]

Most surgeons will use packing at the end of the procedure to stent the meatus open. Resorbable and nonresorbable materials have been used. Gelfoam (Pfizer, New York, NY) (absorbable gelatin sponge) can be placed in the medial end of the cavity to hold the tympanomeatal flap and tympanic membrane grafts in place. Gelfoam can usually be easily removed with suction or alligator forceps in the postoperative period, even in children, or it can be left in place to dissolve

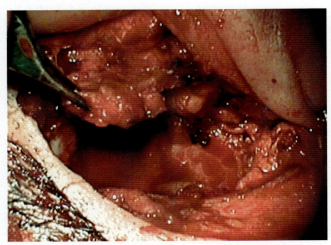

Fig. 5.10 The conchomeatal flap is pulled backward. In this example, the subcutaneous tissue of the conchomeatal flap is preserved so that a fibromuscular (Palva) flap results. By placing stay sutures in the midportion of the flap and turning this fibrous tissue into the posterior aspect of the cavity, a partial obliteration can be achieved.

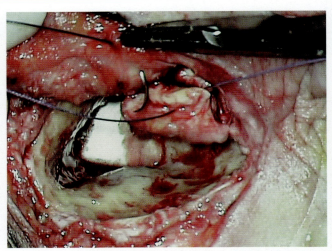

Fig. 5.11 Stay sutures are placed between the conchomeatal skin and the conchal perichondrium, so that the meatus will remain open.

gradually. Bacitracin ointment can also be placed at the base of the cavity, although it will liquefy more quickly than Gelfoam. Merogel (Medtronic Corp., Mystic, CT) (derived from hyaluronic acid) has also been adapted for this purpose. Nonresorbable packing materials include thin silicone sheeting, Owen's silk, or expandable sponges (eg, Merocel, Medtronic Corp.). A rosebud packing can be fashioned and filled with Gelfoam, antibiotic-impregnated gauze, or cottonoid discs. Our own preference is to use Gelfoam medially, followed by a thick cushion of bacitracin ointment, and to fold a strip of Xeroform gauze (Covidien, Mansfield, MA) into the meatus. The Xeroform layer is bacteriostatic and nonadherent and can usually be removed painlessly and without difficulty at the first postoperative visit. The remaining Gelfoam and bacitracin ointment can be gently suctioned or simply left to dissolve.

The packing is removed at 7 to 10 days postoperative. The patient is started on antibiotic eardrops (eg, ofloxacin solu-

tion, 4 drops twice a day), and told to keep the ear dry. If granulation tissue forms in the zone between the skin edges, it can be lightly cauterized with topical silver nitrate. Polypoid granulation tissue can be debrided after cauterizing its base. By 4 to 6 weeks postoperative, a large, stable meatus usually results (**Fig. 5.12**).

◆ External Canal Cholesteatoma and Keratosis Obturans

External canal cholesteatoma is much less common than cholesteatoma of the middle ear and mastoid. This lesion typically presents with otorrhea and chronic, dull pain from local invasion into the bony EAC. Clinically, it has the same appear-

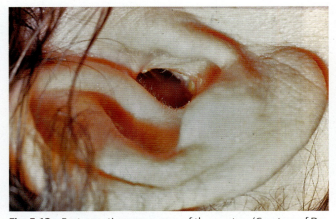

Fig. 5.12 Postoperative appearance of the meatus. (Courtesy of Dr. Simon Parisier.)

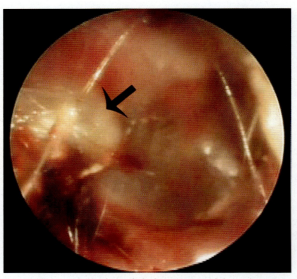

Fig. 5.13 An external canal cholesteatoma of the right ear, appearing as a pearlescent lesion (*arrow*) with adjacent inflammation and ulceration of the skin of the floor of the ear canal.

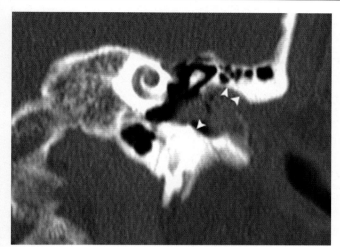

Fig. 5.14 Computed tomographic scan, in coronal plane, showing keratosis obturans. The soft tissue lesion has filled and widened the bony canal (*arrowheads*), without causing bone necrosis.

ance as middle ear cholesteatoma, a pearlescent ball of skin, often with surrounding inflammation or granulation tissue (**Fig. 5.13**). External canal cholesteatoma always involves the inferior aspect of the ear canal, although it may grow to fill the entire canal.[9] On computed tomographic (CT) imaging, bony erosion of the floor of the ear canal will usually be seen.[10]

Primary and secondary forms have been identified. The primary form is idiopathic, although there is evidence that repeated minor trauma inflicted by the patient might be necessary for its formation. The secondary form is usually due to obstruction of the canal (eg, by a bony osteoma) or to focal injury of the EAC by prior surgery or radiation. Very occasionally, a middle ear cholesteatoma will grow exophytically into the EAC; this should not be mistaken for an EAC cholesteatoma and should be treated according to the principles covered elsewhere in this book.

The treatment of external canal cholesteatoma is wide surgical excision of the lesion with a cuff of normal skin.[9,11] The bone is then recontoured with a diamond burr, attempting to avoid opening the mastoid air cells. A split-thickness skin graft may be applied for soft tissue coverage if a significant area of exposed bone remains.

Keratosis obturans is a similar but separate condition. Keratosis obturans is a plug of cerumen and keratin that occludes the entire ear canal, and that causes widening of the bony EAC. In contrast to EAC cholesteatoma, which begins in the inferior part of the bony EAC, keratosis involves the entire circumference of the ear canal, and it is frequently bilateral. It occurs in younger patients, and is associated with sinusitis and bronchiectasis. It presents with painful occlusion and hearing loss.[12,13] CT will reveal a nonerosive soft tissue lesion with circumferential bony expansion of the EAC (**Fig. 5.14**). The absence of bone necrosis and skin ulceration are the most important features that distinguish keratosis obturans from EAC cholesteatoma.[14]

This condition is treated by complete removal of the abnormal plug by curettage, which may require local anesthetic injection (or general anesthesia in children or uncooperative adults), followed by recleaning every few months to prevent reaccumulation. Keratosis obturans will tend to recur if left unattended.

References

1. Paparella MM, Meyerhoff WL. "How I do it"—otology and neurology: a specific issue and its solution. Meatoplasty. Laryngoscope 1978;88(2 Pt 1):357–359
2. Lempert J. Lempert endaural subcortical mastoidotympanectomy for the cure of chronic persistent suppurative otitis media. Arch Otolaryngol 1949;49(1):20–35
3. Raut VV, Rutka JA. The Toronto meatoplasty: enhancing one's results in canal wall down procedures. Laryngoscope 2002;112(11):2093–2095
4. Eisenman DJ, Parisier SC. Meatoplasty: the cartilage of the floor of the ear canal. Laryngoscope 1999;109(5):840–842
5. Saunders JE, Shoemaker DL, McElveen JT Jr. Reconstruction of the radical mastoid. Am J Otol 1992;13(5):465–469
6. Donaldson JA, Duckert LG. "How I do it"—otology and neurotology: a specific issue and its solution. Meatoplasty. Laryngoscope 1981;91(10):1757–1758
7. Fagan P, Ajal M. Z-meatoplasty of the external auditory canal. Laryngoscope 1998;108(9):1421–1422
8. Mirck PG. The M-meatoplasty of the external auditory canal. Laryngoscope 1996;106(3 Pt 1):367–369
9. Dubach P, Häusler R. External auditory canal cholesteatoma: reassessment of and amendments to its categorization, pathogenesis, and treatment in 34 patients. Otol Neurotol 2008;29(7):941–948
10. Heilbrun ME, Salzman KL, Glastonbury CM, Harnsberger HR, Kennedy RJ, Shelton C. External auditory canal cholesteatoma: clinical and imaging spectrum. AJNR Am J Neuroradiol 2003;24(4):751–756
11. Lin YS. Surgical results of external canal cholesteatoma. Acta Otolaryngol 2009;129(6):615–623
12. Sismanis A, Huang CE, Abedi E, Williams GH. External ear canal cholesteatoma. Am J Otol 1986;7(2):126–129
13. Piepergerdes MC, Kramer BM, Behnke EE. Keratosis obturans and external auditory canal cholesteatoma. Laryngoscope 1980;90(3):383–391
14. Persaud RA, Hajioff D, Thevasagayam MS, Wareing MJ, Wright A. Keratosis obturans and external ear canal cholesteatoma: how and why we should distinguish between these conditions. Clin Otolaryngol Allied Sci 2004;29(6):577–581

6

Situations That Arise at Surgery: Anatomical Issues

This chapter addresses the unique situations that arise during cholesteatoma surgery. Some of the surgical tactics described herewith will depend on a surgeon's skill and experience. The goals of surgery may vary depending on the situation created by the cholesteatoma, but in general they are either to completely remove the cholesteatoma or to exteriorize the cholesteatoma, making a safe ear amenable to trouble-free postoperative assessment and cleaning. The preservation or restoration of hearing function is a second key goal, which may sometimes be accomplished in a single operation, or as a planned second-stage surgery.

The unique biological behavior of cholesteatoma and the intricate anatomy of the temporal bone create challenges during surgery. These situations are discussed individually or together. In this chapter we will address some of the more common anatomical situations that may arise. These include disease on the oval window; disease in the sinus tympani (the most frequent site for recurrence); disease on the bare facial nerve; lateral semicircular canal fistula; cholesteatosis/giant cholesteatoma; and cerebrospinal fluid (CSF) leakage/encephalocele. In the next chapter, we will discuss hearing issues that arise at surgery, namely, intact ossicular chain, disease in the normal, better, or only-hearing ear, and bilateral cholesteatoma.

◆ Oval Window Disease

Dissecting disease from the stapes and oval window is a common event at surgery. Cholesteatoma in the middle ear can insinuate itself in and around the stapes. This is particularly true of retraction pocket cholesteatoma of the pars tensa that forms in the posterosuperior quadrant and travels medially toward the promontory and posteriorly into the sinus tympani. The stapes superstructure and lenticular process are contained within a mucosal envelope that can act as a conduit for the vertical spread of disease from the tympanic membrane to the promontory (**Fig. 6.1**).[1] Attic cholesteatoma can also involve the stapes by growing medially from

the posterior epitympanic space along the long process of the incus.

Surgical access to cholesteatoma of the middle ear is gained through the external ear canal and medial to the remainder of the tympanic membrane when intact. Surgical dissection around the stapes is best approached in a stepwise, superior to inferior direction (**Fig. 6.2A**). If the long process of the incus is still intact, it can be followed inferiorly and sometimes preserved. If the lenticular process of the incus has been eroded (a common occurrence), the incus can be lifted laterally or, if necessary, removed for better exposure. This is necessary when disease extends into the attic in the plane medial to the incus. Once the incus is fully disarticulated, curettage of

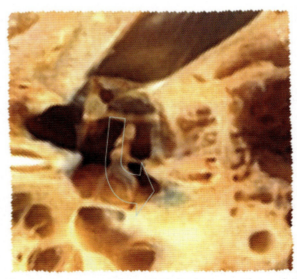

Fig. 6.1 Pars tensa cholesteatomas begin as retraction pockets in the posterosuperior quadrant and travel medially toward the promontory and posteriorly into the sinus tympani. The stapes superstructure and lenticular process act as a conduit for the spread of disease from the tympanic membrane to the promontory.

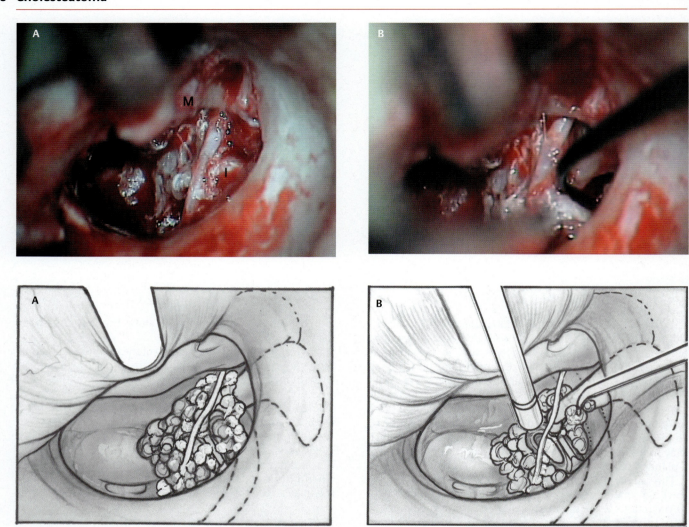

Fig. 6.2 Dissection of a left middle ear cholesteatoma from the stapes, left ear. **(A)** Cholesteatoma enveloping stapes. M, malleus; I, incus, eroded. **(B)** Dissection proceeds in a downward direction, exposing eroded incus, and freeing disease from capitulum while stabilizing crura with suction.

the scutum provides access to the epitympanum, which facilitates removal of the incus. Cholesteatoma that extends superiorly will require an atticotomy to access the disease.

The stapes can be difficult to identify visually when it is covered or encased by granulation tissue and cholesteatoma. Gentle palpation should be performed to locate the superstructure before lifting the cholesteatoma from this area. In some instances, the stapes may be deflected inferiorly toward the promontory and can be unintentionally fractured or mobilized if this is not recognized. Once the stapes head is identified by palpation and inspection, disease can be peeled off the crura in medial-to-lateral and posterior-to-anterior directions using the trailing edge of a sharp pick (**Fig. 6.2B–D**). The stapedial tendon is often present and provides countertraction during the posterior to anterior dissection. The side of a 3F Baron suction tip can be used to steady the crura during this maneuver. The matrix can then be sharply dissected off the footplate and from between the crura. This maneuver requires pa-

tience and a steady hand. If this proves to be difficult, raising concern that continued dissection may lead to stapes mobilization and extraction, consideration should be given toward staging the procedure and returning at a future date.

Occasionally the crura are eroded and may become dislocated from the footplate.[2] Using a sweeping motion will ensure that the crura are not forcibly broken because the footplate may then fracture or become mobilized. If a perilymph leak does develop through a fractured footplate or a torn annular ligament, it should be immediately covered with a graft of fascia or areolar tissue. Traumatic luxation of the stapes can result in vertigo and permanent sensorineural hearing loss, and so this aspect of the dissection must be done with great care.[3–5]

Not uncommonly, the entire superstructure will have been eroded by the disease, and the matrix will be adherent to the footplate. Complete removal can be difficult because the defined matrix layer is often lacking in this location, and

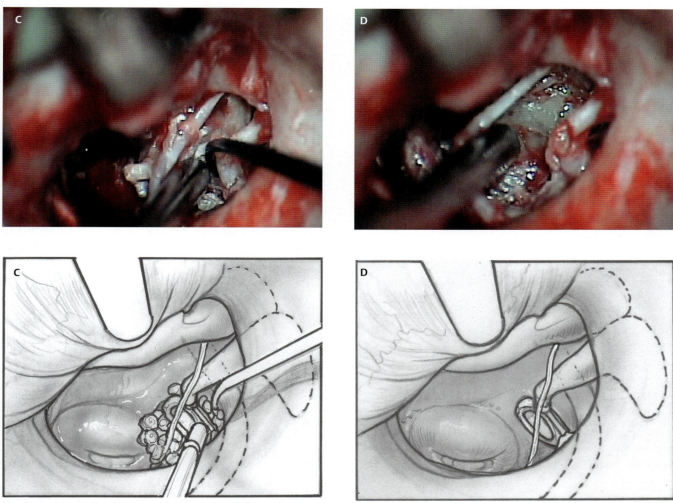

Fig. 6.2 (*Continued*) **(C)** Matrix is then peeled away from inferior aspect of crura. **(D)** Completed dissection.

the footplate may be covered with inflammatory granulation tissue.[2] In these cases, applying firm but gentle pressure with the tip of a curved needle or hockey stick (whirlybird) dissector will allow an edge of the matrix to be elevated off the stapes footplate, still working in a superior to inferior direction. If the matrix breaks apart, the same technique is used but the disease will be delivered piecemeal. It is important not to leave residual matrix in the sulcus between the oval window and the facial nerve.

It should be noted that the intact canal wall mastoidectomy with facial recess usually allows sufficient access to the anterior sinus tympani for dissection of disease, especially when the diseased incus is removed and the incus buttress is taken down; but there will be a few surgical situations when exposure is limited because the sinus tympani extends medial to the facial nerve. When the facial recess approach is not enough, the surgeon may enlarge the external ear canal medially by the annulus gaining exposure to the sinus tympani space through the ear canal. It may be necessary to sacrifice the chorda tympani nerve, which would be done anyway with the canal wall down alternative.

If additional exposure to the sinus tympani is needed, the canal wall down approach provides a less encumbered view of the oval window and better access to the sinus tympani. From the surgeon's vantage point—looking from the mastoid toward the middle ear—the lateral semicircular canal, facial nerve, and stapes fall in a line and lie at the same depth (**Fig. 6.3A,B**). The lateral semicircular canal is the most consistent landmark, located at the base of the mastoid antrum. Cholesteatoma matrix should be lifted off the dome of the lateral canal, working in a posterior-to-anterior direction from the antrum toward the middle ear. Once the dense ivory bone of the lateral semicircular canal is exposed, the matrix is peeled away from the lateral aspect of the facial nerve, looking carefully for any dehiscence and avoiding pressure from the instrument against the facial nerve. The sulcus between the facial nerve (fallopian canal) and the lip of the oval window forms an acute angle, so the surgeon should not disrupt the matrix in this area. The disease should then be lifted off the stapes superstructure, taking care not to rock the stapes excessively (**Fig. 6.4**). Finding the superstructure may be tricky—it may be covered by disease, displaced inferiorly, or

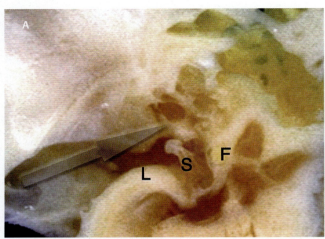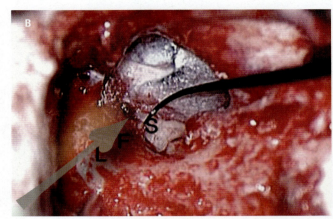

Fig. 6.3 **(A)** The lateral semicircular canal (L), facial nerve (F), and stapes (S) lie at the same depth and in a straight line, as shown in this cross-sectional view of a cadaver temporal bone, and in **(B)** a surgical photograph of a left ear mastoidectomy. The surgeon's line of sight is shown (*arrow*) when looking from the mastoid toward the middle ear.

absent—but it can usually be located by palpating through the matrix with a pick, stripping disease from posterior to anterior using a cupped forceps or sharply cutting away the inflammatory/cholesteatoma mass with a fine microscissors. The pyramidal process can be a good landmark for finding the stapes in disease; it transmits the stapedius tendon that attaches to the posterior crus of the stapes. Once the superstructure is located, the disease can be dissected off, working from the base of the posterior crus toward the capitulum,

while stabilizing the crura with a suction (**Fig. 6.4**). The stapes crura may be eroded, and the superstructure can occasionally become detached from the footplate during the dissection. Sometimes erosion of the crura will not be apparent until after they are exposed.

In canal wall up surgery, the entire oval window is not as easy to expose. A purely transcanal, trans–middle ear approach can be used, but if the disease extends back toward the sinus tympani or superiorly toward the attic the bony canal will have to be widened. If a mastoidectomy is done first, a transmastoid atticotomy plus facial recess approach will provide exposure to the posterior middle ear and give better access to the sinus tympani. The route to the oval window through the facial recess is the same as in canal wall down. However, the angle of visualization is more acute from the perspective of the mastoid. Again, the lateral semicircular canal, facial nerve, and stapes fall in a line. In most cases, when disease is present in the posterior epitympanic space, the incus will have to be removed. It is important to thin the posterior bony canal wall to its cortical layer with a diamond drill so as to gain exposure as anteriorly as possible. It is useful when drilling to conceptualize the shape of the bony canal wall as a truncated cone rather than a cylinder. The incus buttress can be maintained, but more often it is helpful to drill it away, allowing better access to the area around the stapes. In these surgical situations, the incus is frequently eroded, justifying removal of the diseased incus. If the incudostapedial joint is still intact it should be disarticulated and the incus pushed superiorly into the attic. In canal wall up surgery, the strategy should be to mobilize the matrix from behind forward, dissecting it off the lateral canal and facial nerve superiorly, and out of the sinus tympani posteriorly, toward the stapes superstructure.

By rotating the operating table toward the surgeon, the middle ear dissection can be accomplished through the ear canal. In difficult cases, it may be necessary to leave matrix

Fig. 6.4 Cholesteatoma matrix on stapes superstructure, right ear. The stapes is steadied with a 3F Baron suction tip. A Rosen needle is used to lift the matrix off the superstructure, working in a medial-to-lateral direction.

attached to the footplate. With this situation, Silastic sheeting can be placed in the middle ear and the tympanic membrane grafted. At the second stage, the cholesteatoma (frequently a pearl remnant) is resected, then a footplate to malleus or footplate to tympanic membrane (type V) reconstruction is performed. Alternatively, it may be necessary to leave matrix attached to the footplate. This situation requires that the middle ear be left open, and a second procedure is done at a later stage to remove the residual.

Ossicular reconstruction can be performed after removing disease from the footplate, provided the surgeon is confident that there is no residual disease. A partial prosthesis can be used if the stapes superstructure is intact, or a total prosthesis if the superstructure is absent. Sometimes a total prosthesis can be placed against the footplate between the crura if the superstructure is tenuous or leaning forward, which helps to maintain stability of the prosthesis.

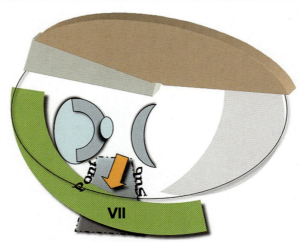

Fig. 6.5 The sinus tympani is illustrated schematically. This space (*arrow*) is bounded superiorly by the ponticulum (Pont) at the level of the oval window, and inferiorly by the subiculum (Sub) at the level of the round window. It travels medial to the facial nerve (VII) as shown.

◆ Sinus Tympani Disease

The sinus tympani, or tympanic sinus, is a triangular space that communicates with the mesotympanum. It is bounded superiorly and inferiorly by two ridges of bone, the ponticulum and subiculum, and laterally by the fallopian canal of the facial nerve. The presence of the facial nerve prevents the sinus tympani from being unroofed, which prohibits complete visualization of its contents. It is often not possible to fully inspect the confines of this space, raising the risk of leaving residual disease. It is important to attempt to keep the entire sac or retraction pocket intact to insure its total removal.

Sinus tympani cholesteatoma arises most often from a retraction pocket of the posterosuperior quadrant of the tympanic membrane, which, when it develops in this area, can grow medialward and become invasive.[6] It is also encountered in attic cholesteatomas that extend downward toward the middle ear, and in middle ear atelectasis, where a retraction pocket can extend into the sinus and be very difficult to remove. A marginal perforation at the posterior annulus may also give rise to keratin matrix that migrates into the sinus tympani.

The anatomy of the sinus tympani is shown in **Fig. 6.5**. The ponticulum, which forms the superior limit, is a bridge of bone found at the level of the inferior lip of the oval window. The subiculum, which forms the inferior boundary, is at the level of the superior lip of the round window. The sinus tympani extends medial to the mastoid segment of the facial nerve. Its size is variable, and it can be quite deep and extensive. A related space, termed the posterior sinus, lies superior to the sinus tympani and just posterior to the stapes. At times this space is contiguous with the sinus tympani, if the ponticulum is rudimentary in size. The anatomy of these spaces has been well demonstrated and beautifully illustrated in recent publications by Holt and Marchioni et al.[7,8]

Disease enters the sinus tympani by migrating medially along the lenticular process and stapes superstructure, then posteriorly along the plane of the promontory. This direction of growth can be appreciated in cases of retraction pockets arising from posterior middle ear collapse (**Fig. 6.6A**).

Surgical access to the sinus tympani is made challenging by the presence of the facial nerve. The sinus can be accessed either through the middle ear via a tympanoplasty approach, enlarging the posterior bony canal and scutum, or through the mastoid via facial recess or canal wall down approaches. Both approaches require that the bone anterior to the facial nerve be thinned aggressively to provide as much exposure as possible. Even so, clearing disease from the apex of the sinus tympani is a partly blind maneuver.

In the tympanoplasty approach, a generous bony canalplasty should be done first, removing bone posteriorly to the mastoid segment of the facial nerve.[9] This is done by saucerizing the posterior canal bone until a large, concave contour results, identifying the facial nerve at the second genu and following it inferiorly. To fashion a round canal, it is necessary to remove additional bone from the inferior and superior canal wall. The latter initiates a transcanal atticotomy. In cases where disease involves the attic and antrum, it may be safer to assure exteriorization performing a canal wall down mastoidectomy.

In the facial recess approach, the facial recess opening must be sufficient to allow maximal visualization as well as to permit instrumentation. This requires creating an adequate vertical opening (~3 mm in height) by thinning the posterior canal wall aggressively, at least up to the chorda tympani, and sometimes transecting the chorda to expose the fibrous annulus. The facial nerve should then be skeletonized and the bony ledge anterior to the nerve removed as well (**Fig. 6.6B**). This requires using a diamond burr to define the circumference of the nerve, as previously discussed in Chapter 4. Sometimes the pyramidal process will also need to be removed. Once the bony approach is completed, the patient's head can be tilted (by airplaning the operating table) so as to gain the best possible view into the sinus. Because the facial nerve is the limit-

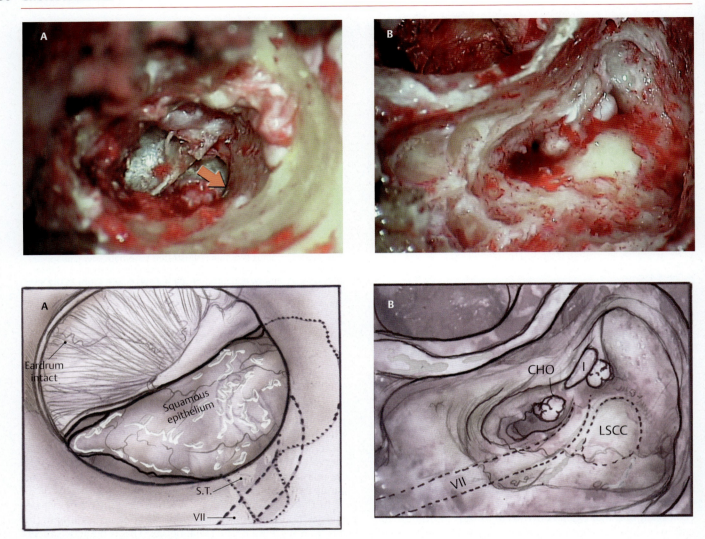

Fig. 6.6 Dissection of a cholesteatoma from the sinus tympani via the facial recess, left ear. **(A)** Middle ear cholesteatoma viewed through the ear canal, extending posteriorly toward the sinus tympani (*arrow*). **(B)** Mastoidectomy with a facial recess approach exposes the posterior limit of the cholesteatoma sac.

ing factor, the exposure obtained through the facial recess approach should be similar to the transcanal approach already described (**Fig. 6.6C**). If still greater access is needed, the canal wall should be taken down, initially to the chorda tympani inlet; and if this does not provide enough exposure then the canal wall is taken down to the level of the facial nerve.

Once adequate surgical exposure is obtained, the disease can be dissected using blunt right angle instruments. A whirlybird dissector (equivalent to the Hough excavator) or Derlacki elevator is well suited for this task. The object is to create a plane between the bone and the outside of the epithelial capsule to deliver the sac in toto. The matrix should be held together as a shell if possible (**Fig. 6.7A,B**). Piecemeal dissection should be avoided. If the capsule starts to break, a

new point of dissection should be started. If the sac cannot be held together, then the debris should be evacuated, and a peeling action should be used to deliver the sac.

A mirror or endoscope is very helpful to inspect the sinus tympani after dissection to ascertain that no residual disease remains (**Fig. 6.6D**). Residual cholesteatoma has a pearlescent appearance and is usually easy to discern from mucosa. A mirror is simpler to set up than an endoscope because the microscope does not have to be moved; however, it is tricky to use and requires a bit of practice. The otoendoscope has gained increasing attention for enhanced visualization to facilitate complete removal of sinus tympani disease.[10] The endoscope offers the benefit of superb optics and provides a panoramic view, allowing eradication of the cholesteatoma, often through a purely transcanal approach. The endoscope

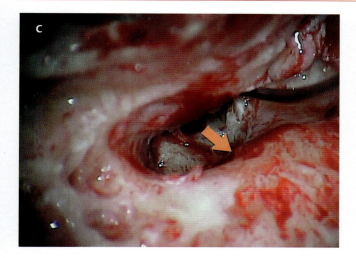

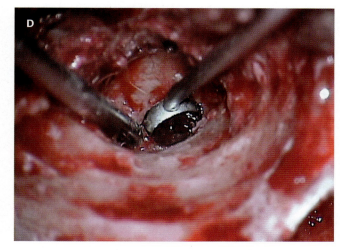

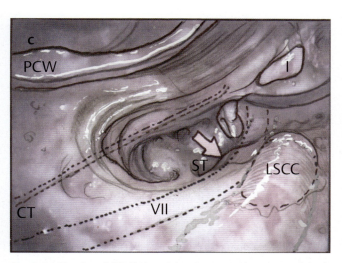

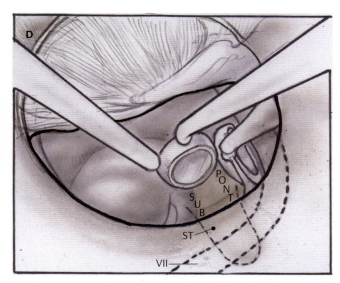

Fig. 6.6 (*Continued*) **(C)** Skeletonizing the mastoid segment of the facial nerve allows access to the sinus tympani (*arrow*). **(D)** After dissecting the sac from the sinus tympani, a mirror is used to confirm that there is no residual disease.

requires a modification of technique, where the scope must be steadied during the surgical dissection. If the operating surgeon holds the endoscope while viewing the TV monitor, only one hand is available for surgical dissection. An alternative method requires two sets of hands as well as access from both sides of the operating table. When using the endoscope, care must be taken to avoid traumatizing the stapes crura. The instrument is compromised by the presence of blood given that it may be difficult to navigate a suction tip into the sinus cavity. Chemical defogging agents are also generally needed.

In cases of very deep sinus tympani, a retrofacial approach has been proposed. This requires complete circumferential skeletonization of the nerve and a superior angle of drilling. This approach should only rarely be needed.[11]

Cases of middle ear atelectasis with sinus tympani retraction pockets are particularly difficult to manage. Because the sac is empty, it can fragment easily requiring great care and patience to remove the sac completely. Leonetti et al have reported on a technique of exteriorizing the sinus tympani and dissecting the sac in toto in a series of cases, with very good control over long-term follow-up.[12,13] The technique they describe requires that a myringotomy tube be maintained long term to prevent re-formation of the sac.

Tympanic Membrane Cholesteatoma

Tympanic membrane cholesteatoma is a special situation that may arise during surgery and is occasionally unexpected by

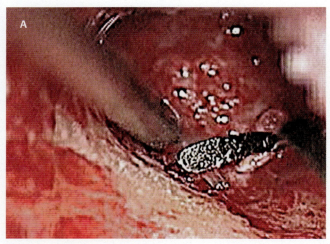

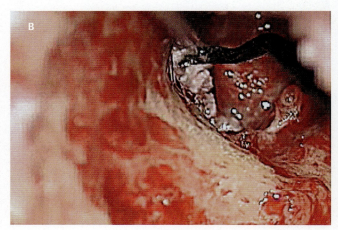

Fig. 6.7 Dissection of sinus tympani via transcanal approach, right ear. **(A)** A whirlybird dissector is inserted into the sinus. **(B)** The sinus contents are delivered using a sweeping motion to separate the sac from the bone.

the surgeon. In the office, a perforation may be noticed with a whitish discoloration of the remaining tympanic membrane. On first otoscopic examination, one may believe that this is tympanic membrane tympanosclerosis. Occasionally, there may be migratory epithelium as seen in the figure, which will alert the surgeon to the presence of this same type of migratory epithelium on the undersurface of the tympanic membrane (**Fig. 6.8A,B**).

The usual approach to tympanic membrane surgery is undertaken. When the tympanomeatal flap is elevated, the undersurface of the tympanic membrane is found to have a thin layer of squamous epithelium lacing the medial layer. Occasionally there may be free cholesteatoma in the middle ear and on the promontory. The epithelial matrix may extend along the tympanic membrane to the fibrous annulus and onto the mucosal layer of the middle ear cleft. The matrix may also wrap around the malleus and tensor tympani muscle. A 30-degree telescope is useful to inspect the undersurface of the tympanic membrane to define the extent of involvement.

The operation must eradicate the disease and may need to be quite extensive. If the malleus and tensor muscle are involved, then the surgeon must remove most of the tympanic membrane and perform either an underlay or over–under tympanoplasty to make certain of total removal of this process. It may even be necessary to disarticulate the incudostapedial joint to gain enough access to totally remove the epithelial matrix around the malleus and tensor muscle. Ossicular reconstruction with an incus interposition graft is then performed. Close patient follow- up is necessary for years to make sure there is no recurrence.

◆ Collapsed Middle Ear Space

Posterior collapse of the tympanic membrane that reduces the middle ear space presents a challenge. Many times one will find a contracted middle ear space where the annulus is closer to the promontory (especially inferiorly) than in other

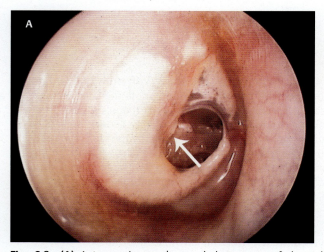

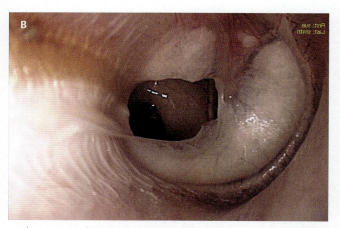

Fig. 6.8 **(A)** A tympanic membrane cholesteatoma of the right ear. The sac can be seen protruding through the perforation (*arrow*). **(B)** It can be mistaken for tympanosclerosis, a common benign finding. Eradication of the disease requires removing and regrafting the involved area of the tympanic membrane, in addition to removing the disease from the middle ear space.

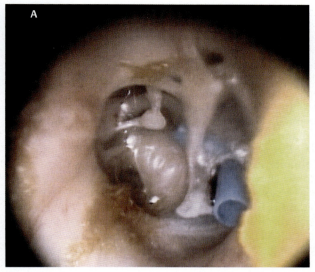

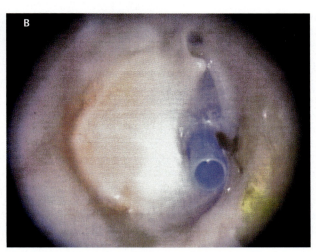

Fig. 6.9 Posterior tympanic membrane collapse can coexist with a pneumatized anterior middle ear space. **(A)** A severely retracted tympanic membrane in the right ear of an 11-year-old boy with normal hearing. A tympanostomy tube failed to provide any pneumatization to the posterior middle ear space. **(B)** At surgery, the drum epithelium was separated from the promontory mucosa and a cartilage tympanoplasty was done, reconstituting the middle ear space.

diseased ears. Dissecting the squamous epithelium from the oval window, sinus tympani, and round window is difficult to do without leaving disease behind, as discussed in the previous sections. Creating and maintaining a pneumatized middle ear space is an additional challenge because a severely retracted tympanic membrane (or narrow middle ear cleft) has the propensity to re-retract over time. A tympanostomy tube will probably not correct the problem once middle ear adhesions have formed (**Fig. 6.9A**).

There are two possible ways to deal with a collapsed middle ear space—either the tympanic membrane can be elevated and the middle ear space reconstituted with or without an intact canal wall mastoidectomy,[14] or a canal wall down mastoidectomy can be performed, exteriorizing the disease process. Preoperatively, an estimate can be made of the potential for reconstituting the middle ear space by trying to lift the tympanic membrane away from the promontory with pneumatic otoscopy or by having the patient perform a forceful Valsalva maneuver. It is helpful to judge whether there is aeration anterior to the malleus—if so, it is possible that the posterior disease is old and there is now adequate eustachian tube function. Even in patients with complete atelectasis of the tympanic membrane, eustachian tube function may still be adequate to re-create an aerated middle ear space, provided that the patient does not have severe allergies, gastroesophageal reflux, history of smoking, sleep apnea, or severe nasal and sinus disease.

If the middle ear can be partially or totally inflated, then one can perform a tympanoplasty (with or without an intact canal wall mastoidectomy), placing one or two sheets of medium-thick silicone (Silastic) sheeting on the promontory to maintain the space.[15] When this is done in conjunction with a canal wall up mastoidectomy, the Silastic sheeting can be placed through the facial recess. Cartilage may be a better grafting material than fascia in these cases because it provides stiffness and

greater resistance to retraction (**Fig. 6.9B**).[16] If there is erosion of the incus and stapes superstructure, an ossiculoplasty with a total replacement prosthesis can be performed at the same time. If the superstructure is present, a partial replacement prosthesis can be used or the drum or graft can be attached directly to the stapes head ("myringostapediopexy," or type III ossicular reconstruction). In the short term, a ventilating tube may be helpful to prevent recurrent middle ear collapse,[17] but if a cartilage tympanoplasty is done this may not be necessary.[18]

In many cases, however, the tympanic membrane will be firmly adherent to the promontory mucosa and the middle ear space cannot be re-created. In such a situation, it is better to leave the tympanic membrane epithelium in place and perform a canal wall down (modified radical) mastoidectomy or atticotomy (in a mastoid with limited pneumatization) so as

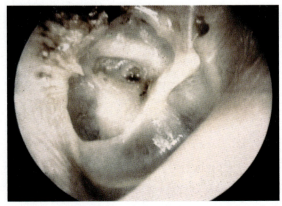

Fig. 6.10 A retraction pocket cholesteatoma of the right ear that has eroded the incus and stapes superstructure and become adherent to the promontory, stapes footplate, and facial nerve. In this case, it was impossible to separate the drum from the promontory so a canal wall down mastoidectomy was done, without ossicular reconstruction.

to exteriorize the disease (**Fig. 6.10**). This will have the effect of creating an open cavity with a lower chance of recurrence. Middle ear function will be compromised, but the tympanic membrane will remain stable in this position over time. Hearing results will result in a moderate air–bone gap, but a maximum conductive hearing loss may be avoided if there is isolation between the round window and oval window by having the tympanic membrane tented over the promontory leaving a residual air space over the round window (this is known as a *cavum minor* or type IV ossicular reconstruction).

The technique of re-creating a middle ear is illustrated here. At surgery, the ear is first inspected, and a suction can be used to assess whether the tympanic membrane is adherent to the promontory mucosa (**Fig. 6.11A**). The tympanomeatal flap is elevated up to the fibrous annulus. The tympanic membrane epithelium will travel medial and posterior to the bony annulus and can be difficult to separate. One should try to find a pocket of pneumatization to begin

dissection. This can often be found inferiorly toward the hypotympanum or anteriorly at the eustachian tube entrance. Curetting the bony annulus is helpful to gain exposure in the posterior mesotympanum. Care should be taken not to tear the flap because the thin epithelium will be difficult to retrieve from the posterior middle ear space once it becomes separated. The technique requires a curved (Rosen) needle or right angle dissector, delicate technique, and patience. Once the middle ear space is entered, the sac is bluntly dissected from the annulus, working posteriorly toward the sinus tympani (**Fig. 6.11B**). One should attempt to remove disease in continuity from this area. If the disease tracks posteriorly into the sinus tympani, a canal wall up mastoidectomy with facial recess may be necessary to gain adequate exposure (**Fig. 6.11C**). Dissection is continued anteriorly and superiorly, separating the tympanic membrane from the promontory while attempting to leave an intact layer of mucosa (*tympanolysis*).

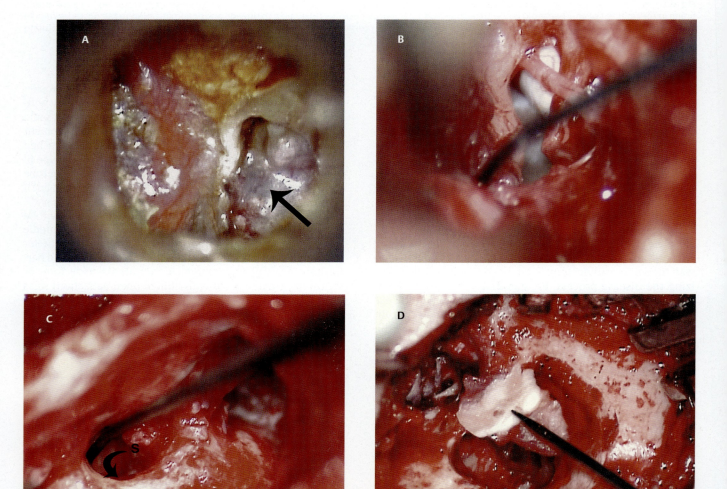

Fig. 6.11 **(A)** A mesotympanic cholesteatoma, left ear, with collapse of the posterior middle ear space (*arrow*). **(B)** The annulus is elevated and the sac is dissected away from the incus/stapes and middle ear promontory. **(C)** The sinus tympani (S) is accessed through the facial recess (VII, facial nerve). **(D)** A cartilage graft is used to reconstruct the tympanic membrane so as to prevent further retraction.

The resulting flap will be thin, and there will be redundant epithelium. An underlay graft of cartilage, taken from the tragus, cimbum, or cavum concha can be used to repair the tympanic membrane and to provide some stiffness (**Fig. 6.11D**). Silastic sheeting can be placed on the promontory to prevent recurrent adhesions. If a mastoidectomy is required, a canal wall up procedure with facial recess should be performed. In that case, the Silastic can be placed over the promontory with an extension of it going through the facial recess. Despite this being a staged procedure with the intention of returning to remove the Silastic, the interim hearing results may be surprisingly good due to conduction of sound energy through the Silastic on the stapes.

The status of the stapes determines the alternatives for ossicular reconstruction. If the superstructure is eroded attempts should be directed toward removing disease off the footplate. Ossicular reconstruction using sculpted incus interposition or total prosthesis can then be performed. If the superstructure is present, the matrix is dissected off the crura using a meticulous and careful technique. If disease is very adherent to the crura, sharp dissection should be used to remove it, or a potassium titanyl phosphate (KTP) or argon laser can be used to vaporize the disease. If the tympanic membrane is attached to the stapes head but not the crura, it can be left intact as a type III reconstruction (myringostapediopexy). Placing an interface of cartilage between the tympanic membrane and head of the stapes provides a greater surface area for transmission of sound vibrations. If there is no pneumatization and no possibility of separating the tympanic membrane from the stapes footplate, then a canal wall down (modified radical) mastoidectomy with type IV tympanoplasty (cavum minor) can be performed.

There is a risk that a retraction pocket may re-form after surgery. If recurrent retraction develops, one should consider inserting a small ventilating tube. This can usually be done postoperatively in the office. Alternatively, a subannular ventilating tube can be placed at the original surgery to provide long-term ventilation.

◆ Dehiscent Facial Nerve Canal

In both attic and middle ear cholesteatomas, the matrix is frequently found covering the tympanic segment of the facial nerve. Familiarity with the anatomy of the nerve in the temporal bone is essential because its position must be anticipated before removing the soft tissue overlying it. Live intraoperative facial nerve monitoring and stimulation are helpful but are not a substitute for anatomical knowledge or proper technique. The facial nerve normally has a thin bony covering (fallopian canal), which is dehiscent in at least 15% of cases (the percentage is probably higher in cholesteatoma because of its erosive nature).[19-22] These dehiscences usually occur along the inferior aspect of the nerve superior to the stapes but may often involve the dorsum of the nerve between the processus cochleariformis and second genu. The processus is an excellent landmark for locating the tympanic segment of the nerve before exposing it. Knowledge of the anticipated location of the facial nerve dehiscence is key to avoiding surgical injury to the nerve.

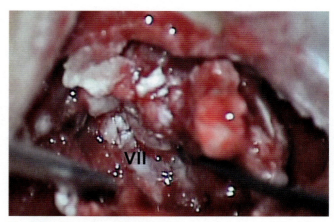

Fig. 6.12 Dissection of disease off the bare facial nerve (VII), right ear. The patient had a facial paralysis 1 month prior to surgery that cleared up with antibiotics and steroids. At surgery, a canal wall down mastoidectomy was performed, and the cholesteatoma sac was lifted off the exposed facial nerve in a superior-to-inferior direction using a stimulating instrument.

The facial nerve is best approached in a superior-to-inferior, posterior-to-anterior direction, using the lateral semicircular canal, stapes, and cochleariform process as landmarks. The facial nerve is approached as the sac is dissected off the medial wall of the attic and lateral semicircular canal. In canal wall up surgery, this requires an adequate (transmastoid) atticotomy. The incus and malleus head will usually be lined by or eroded by disease and will need to be removed. The contents of the sac should be decompressed before the sac itself is lifted or peeled off the medial attic wall. By lifting the matrix in a continuous sheet from the medial attic wall toward the dorsum of the nerve, a plane is developed that allows the disease to be lifted cleanly and without pressure or direct contact with the nerve. This maneuver is illustrated in **Fig. 6.12**. Generally a sharp instrument such as a needle dissector is more effective than a blunt excavator for achieving this. In removing cholesteatoma from around the tympanic segment of the facial nerve, the matrix should be swept off the nerve, toward the stapes, without turning the tip of the instrument toward the facial nerve itself.

The technique of safely dissecting disease from an exposed facial nerve becomes familiar as one gains experience. Dehiscence of the bony fallopian canal should be expected along its inferior surface, the most common location of the exposed nerve. At times, the lateral surface or even the entire circumference of the nerve may be dehiscent in the tympanic segment. The safest strategy is to approach the nerve from superior to inferior beginning along the lateral surface, lifting the matrix away from the nerve sheath while attempting to keep the matrix intact. In cases in which the bony canal is dehiscent, the epineurium may be covered by a layer of slightly inflamed mucosa. The corresponding "edema plane" also helps to protect the nerve from being pulled up with the matrix. Again, using the trailing point of a sharp pick allows this to be done safely and efficiently (**Fig. 6.13A,B**).

The enclosed video that illustrates the removal of residual cholesteatoma from a bare facial nerve in a canal wall down cavity demonstrating the concept of the "edema plane."

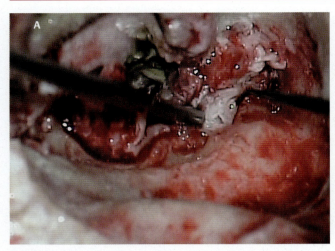
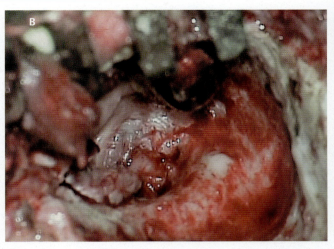

Fig. 6.13 Dissection of disease from the bare facial nerve, left ear. **(A)** The disease is removed working from above downward, using the trailing point of a sharp pick, beginning along the dorsal surface of the nerve. **(B)** The matrix is lifted away from the nerve sheath as an intact layer.

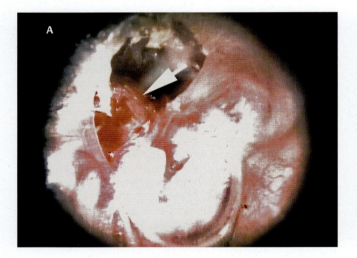
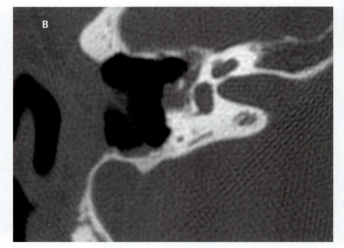

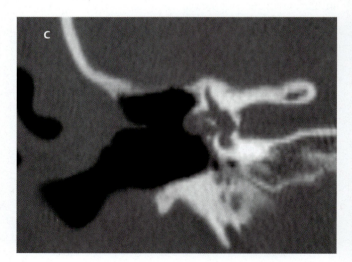

Fig. 6.14 Left ear with recurrent cholesteatoma, preoperative vertigo with tragal pressure. **(A)** Preoperative photograph showing recurrent cholesteatoma (*arrow*) in the middle ear and attic, protruding through the scutum defect. **(B)** Axial computed tomography (CT), showing disease eroding into the lateral semicircular canal. **(C)** Coronal CT, with similar finding.

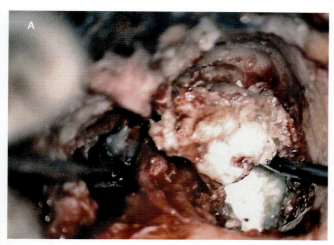

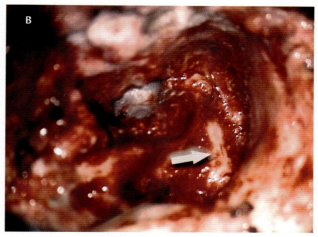

Fig. 6.15 A large recurrent cholesteatoma of the left ear causing a lateral semicircular canal fistula. **(A)** The contents of the sac are being lifted, initially leaving the matrix against the fistula. **(B)** After the matrix is removed, the fistula can be seen (*arrow*). This was immediately covered with fascia, and there was no postoperative change in bone conduction.

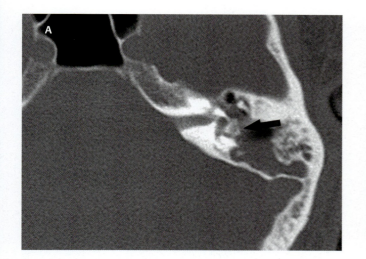

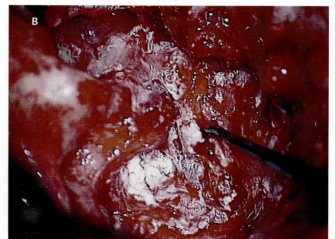

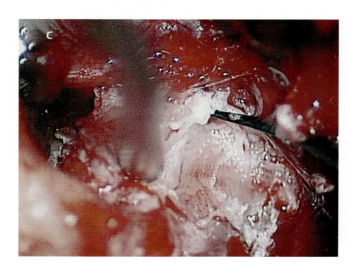

Fig. 6.16 Large cholesteatoma of the left ear with lateral semicircular canal fistula. **(A)** Axial computed tomography showing disease eroding into the lateral semicircular canal (*arrow*). **(B)** Intraoperative photo showing extensive disease. The edge of the matrix is being elevated off the lateral semicircular canal. **(C)** As the matrix is removed, a large area of erosion into the canal lumen is uncovered. The patient developed a *Pseudomonas* infection that resulted in postoperative vertigo and a dead ear.

A facial nerve monitor was in use during the dissection. A stimulating probe tip instrument was also used during this task. Stimulating instruments allow a small electric current (typically 0.05 to 1.0 mA) to be delivered during the critical part of the dissection, giving audible feedback to the surgeon about the proximity of the instrument tip to the bare nerve. Intraoperative facial nerve monitoring and stimulation can be useful adjuncts while dissecting disease off a bare nerve by providing feedback to the surgeon about the location and integrity of the nerve.

The use of routine facial nerve monitoring during surgery of chronic ear disease remains controversial, but its benefit is convincing during a situation such as this one. The monitor can only be effective if it is present and working at the moment that it is needed. There continues to be disagreement about whether the facial nerve monitor should be used routinely and whether its use should constitute the standard of care for surgery of chronic ear disease. This issue is addressed more fully in Chapter 8. It should be remembered that if one encounters questions about the facial nerve dehiscence during surgery, the stimulator-monitor can be connected at that time, testing for nerve integrity prior to continuing facial nerve dissection.

◆ Lateral Semicircular Canal Fistula

Lateral semicircular canal fistula is one of the more common situations encountered during cholesteatoma surgery and is often unrecognized beforehand. Cholesteatoma is an erosive disease. The bony covering of the lateral semicircular canal is susceptible to osteoclasis by the cholesteatoma matrix. Fistulas may be encountered in a significant percentage of cholesteatomas.[23]

The usual presentation of lateral semicircular canal fistula is vertigo, often brought on by the patient sneezing, coughing, spontaneous Valsalva (nose blowing), changing head position, or by pressing on the tragus. The expected clinical finding is a positive fistula test (Politzer sign or Hennebert sign), deviation of the eyes away from the affected ear with positive, or toward the affected ear with negative, pressure in the external canal. The fistula sign can be elicited with the examiner's cupped hand over the external meatus with a pneumatic (Siegle) otoscope or Politzer bag. It should be noted, however, that many lateral semicircular canal fistulas are asymptomatic and are only discovered at surgery. Vertigo may be absent in one third of patients, and the fistula test may be negative 50% of the time.[24] Sensorineural hearing loss may or may not be present.

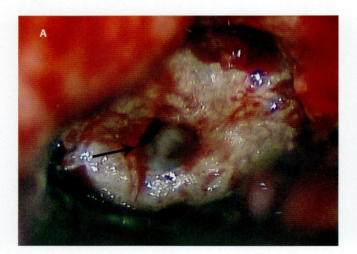

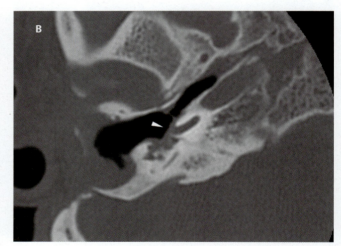

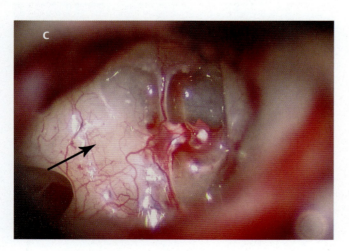

Fig. 6.17 **(A)** A fistula into the cochlea (*arrow*) in a left ear with cholesteatoma. **(B)** A computed tomographic scan showing the area of focal erosion (*arrowhead*). **(C)** Reexploration, 6 months later, showing new bone growth over the area of fistula (*arrow*).

A preoperative computed tomographic (CT) scan is desirable when a fistula is suspected, either by a history of dizziness or by the finding of unilateral sensorineural hearing loss. Erosion of bone is typically observed in the axial images through the plane of the lateral semicircular canal. Fistulas can also be observed in the coronal plane, although an imprecise cut may miss the finding, and volume averaging can give a false-positive finding (**Fig. 6.14A–C**). CT may be falsely negative in 40% of cases.[24]

When a fistula is suspected at surgery, care should be taken to avoid aggressively manipulating disease over the lateral semicircular canal. A canal wall up procedure should be performed initially to debulk the contents of the sac. The matrix should be left over the lateral canal until most of the disease has been removed and the surgeon is ready to deal with the fistula.

How the fistula should be handled remains a matter of debate. Classical teaching maintains that a canal wall down procedure should be done to exteriorize the disease, and a thin layer of matrix should be left in place over the fistula. The residual matrix provides a protective covering for the inner ear, and exteriorization of the cavity limits the potential for infection or continued bone erosion.[25] The residual matrix is used as part of the lining of the new mastoid cavity. If cholesteatoma and granulation tissue are too firmly attached to the matrix to be removed safely, these are better left intact. Postoperative ototopical drops are used with great success to later control this process.

Others have argued for completely removing the matrix over the fistula and resurfacing the labyrinth with fascia, cartilage, or bone pАte. The rationale is to avoid leaving any disease behind, which has the potential for regrowth or reinfection (**Fig. 6.15A,B**).[23,26] It is believed that the inner ear can be safely unroofed without causing permanent loss of cochlear and vestibular function as long as the membra-

nous portion is not violated The evidence for this comes from experimental research on surgical entry into the inner ear,[27] from clinical experience with fenestration surgery for otosclerosis,[26] and, more recently, with posterior semicircular canal occlusion for benign positional vertigo.[28] As a result, some surgeons consider it safe to remove the remaining matrix from over the lateral canal and immediately seal the fistula with autologous material or even bone wax. Some have recommended that this be done in two stages,[29] although the general experience of others suggests that this is not routinely necessary. Kobayashi et al[30] went so far as to advocate that the lateral semicircular canal be intentionally transected, as a method to ablate the canal without creating sensorineural hearing loss. Even with this evidence, we believe it preferable to leave the matrix intact over the fistula whenever there is an infectious component to prevent potential invasion with bacteria.

The results of cholesteatoma surgery in the presence of labyrinthine fistula are generally good, with about an 85% rate of postoperative hearing preservation and a < 10% rate of dead ears.[24] The risk to the hearing appears to be similar whether or not the matrix is removed. Facial nerve exposure may be more common when fistula is present because there is erosive disease nearby.

The long-term results of fistula repair have not been systematically studied or reported. Postoperatively, vertigo and sensitivity to tragal pressure may not disappear because the fistula remains covered by soft tissue and not bone. Vertigo may occur more readily than usual during postoperative cleaning as it does in patients who have had fenestration operations. The ear may be susceptible to delayed sensorineural hearing loss because of labyrinthine sclerosis or because the open area may allow bacterial toxins to enter the inner ear (**Fig. 6.16A–C**). Fistulas may also occur in recurrent cholesteatoma. Hakuba et al[31] presented 25 labyrinthine

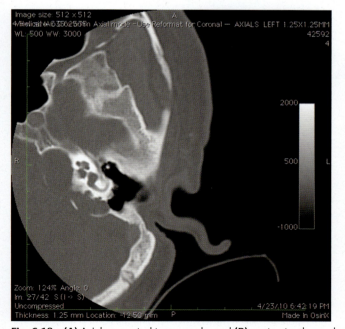

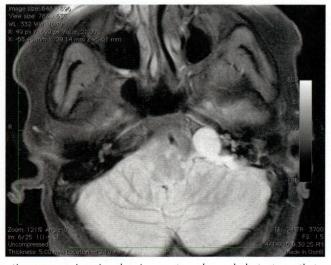

Fig. 6.18 **(A)** Axial computed tomography and **(B)** contrast-enhanced magnetic resonance imaging showing a petrous bone cholesteatoma that required a modified translabyrinthine approach for exteriorization.

fistulae occurring an average of 20 years after canal wall down mastoidectomy surgery. Leaving an open cavity does not guarantee that fistula will never form, especially in patients who have poorly saucerized mastoid cavities. These patients need routine follow-up for years.

Common sense would dictate that labyrinthine fistula be suspected in every case of extensive or recurrent cholesteatoma (since preoperative vertigo is not always present, and CT does not always reveal the fistula). Whenever a fistula is suspected, the lateral semicircular canal should be approached in a careful and controlled manner. The core of the cholesteatoma (debris) should be completely debulked and the matrix removed everywhere except over the lateral semicircular canal. The remaining matrix is then slowly lifted under saline irrigation. If the matrix is unusually adherent or if infection is present, it is wise to leave the matrix intact and perform an open-cavity mastoidectomy. Postoperative antibiotics and steroids may be beneficial in these cases.

Fistulae can also occur into the round or oval windows or by erosion of the promontory. Although these are far less common than lateral semicircular canal fistulae, they can occur nevertheless. Cholesteatoma that has eroded into the vestibule must be either removed completely or exteriorized, even though this has the potential to result in a dead ear. **Figure 6.17** illustrates a case that presented with normal hearing. The cholesteatoma was dissected off the promontory revealing a fistula (**Fig. 6.17A,B**) that was repaired with fascia. Cochlear function was maintained. Six months later, the ear was reexplored for ossicular reconstruction, and the fistula was found to have closed with the new bone (**Fig. 6.17C**).

◆ Cholesteatosis/Giant Cholesteatoma

Giant cholesteatomas are those that occur in well-developed mastoids and replace all the cellular bone. *Cholesteatosis* re-

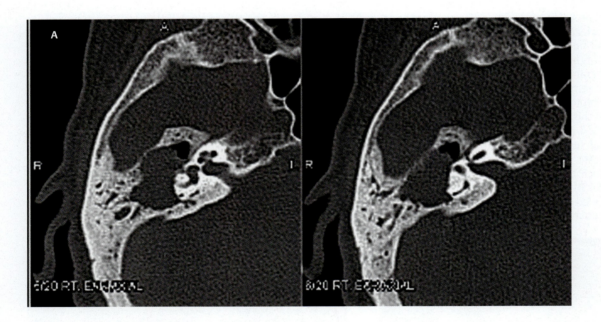

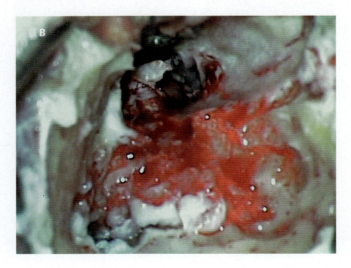

Fig. 6.19 **(A)** Computed tomographic image of a giant cholesteatoma, right ear, filling the mastoid, eroding the cortical bone, and causing a lateral semicircular canal fistula. **(B)** A surgical photo of the lesion, showing extensive involvement and erosion of bone.

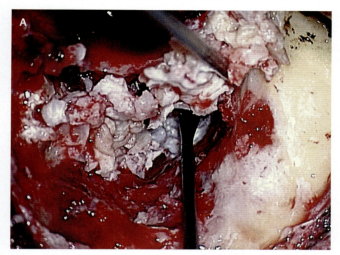 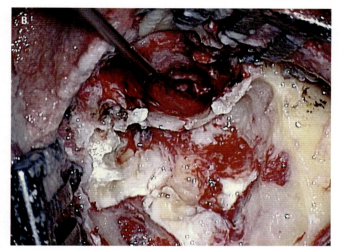

Fig. 6.20 A giant cholesteatoma in a well-developed mastoid cavity, left ear. **(A)** Initial appearance and **(B)** after initial debulking, the lesion is seen to have eroded the facial canal, lateral semicircular canal, and sigmoid sinus plate.

fers to cholesteatoma that burrows into all the pneumatized spaces. *Petrous temporal bone cholesteatoma* is a term given to cholesteatoma that invades or spreads medial to the otic capsule. These are biologically aggressive forms of cholesteatoma that will recur unless they are completely removed. The cause of this aggressive behavior is unknown: these lesions do not differ histologically from routine cholesteatoma. These cholesteatomas can be associated with labyrinthine erosion, facial nerve exposure, dural exposure, and extension to the petrous apex. The surgical procedure will almost always be a canal wall down mastoidectomy (even when the mastoid volume is large) with exenteration of all visible air cell tracts ("subtotal petrosectomy"). Occasionally a translabyrinthine route will be needed to access the petrous apex, or a middle fossa approach to reach the supralabyrinthine tract.[32,33] **Figure 6.18** shows such a case. Preoperative facial nerve paralysis, an exceptionally rare occurrence, may require primary nerve repair with grafting.[33–35] CSF leakage will require primary dural repair. The best strategy to avoid

complications such as these is to create a widely exteriorized cavity with the matrix left intact.

Giant cholesteatomas can develop at any age. In older patients, these may be neglected cholesteatomas that grew to a large size over many years. In younger patients, they may be biologically aggressive lesions that readily erode soft bone. **Figure 6.19A** shows a giant cholesteatoma in an elderly woman. This probably grew insidiously for many years until it reached a large size and was first diagnosed when it became infected. Because of her age, this lesion was initially managed conservatively but eventually required surgery because of persistent infection. The appearance of the ear at surgery is shown in **Fig. 6.19B**.

Figure 6.20A,B shows a giant cholesteatoma in a 40-year-old man who presented with vertigo and purulent otorrhea. He had surprisingly good hearing preoperatively. At surgery, he had extensive disease with profuse green pus, a lateral semicircular canal fistula, and exposed facial nerve. Postoperatively he developed a *Pseudomonas* infection of the

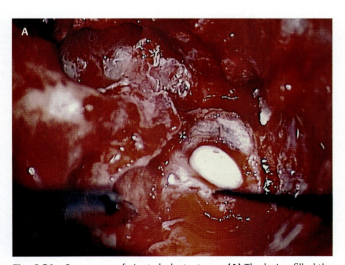 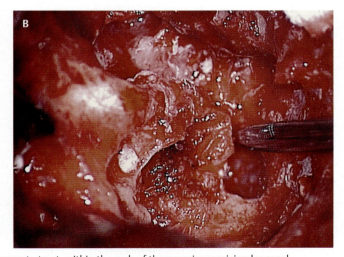

Fig. 6.21 Same case of giant cholesteatoma. **(A)** The lesion filled the subarcuate tract, within the arch of the superior semicircular canal. **(B)** After removal from this area.

mastoid cavity, with suppurative labyrinthitis. He now has a large but stable, dry cavity without evidence of recurrence 3 years postoperatively.

Cholesteatosis is a descriptive term for cholesteatoma that insinuates itself into all the recesses of the temporal bone. It is an aggressive process that occurs in well-developed pneumatized mastoid bones and fortunately is rare. The treatment demands a thorough surgical operation that opens all the involved spaces. This can be a long and arduous procedure. The concept is to remove all the cellular spaces of the mastoid until all that is left is the labyrinth, facial nerve, and tegmen and posterior fossa dural bony plates. This is the procedure that Fisch termed "subtotal petrosectomy." If the disease extends to the petrous apex, it may be impossible to remove entirely without performing a labyrinthectomy as well. **Figure 6.21A,B** shows cholesteatoma pushing through the subarcuate cell tract, between the crura of the superior semicircular canal.

◆ Cerebrospinal Fluid Leak/Encephalocele

CSF leakage is an infrequent occurrence in cholesteatoma surgery. It can occur iatrogenically if the dura is accidentally lacerated, or spontaneously, from a brain herniation (meningoencephalocele) that erodes through its dural covering.

Iatrogenic CSF leaks can occur when drilling near the tegmen, usually when using a cutting burr. The tegmen has an undulating contour, and it is possible to perforate it when skeletonizing its bony surface. The underlying dura is vascular and has a pink appearance when seen through a thin layer of bone. Once exposed, the dural surface will often bleed; the small epidural vessels are easily controlled with bipolar cautery. This epidural bleeding is an important warning to the surgeon because dura will usually withstand one brush with the burr, but not a second one.

Spontaneous tegmen defects are common, occurring in ~20% of temporal bone cadavers, and usually have no serious consequence unless the dura is injured. Cholesteatoma matrix can adhere to bare dura and can be difficult to remove safely (**Fig. 6.22A**). Good technique requires that the margins of the bony tegmen defect first be defined visually. Then the disease can be elevated away from the dura with a blunt dissector using a peeling motion (**Fig. 6.22B**). Blind dissection along the tegmen, on the other hand, may yield an unhappy outcome.

Encephaloceles and meningoceles are herniations of dura with or without brain tissue. The dural covering is often very thin and therefore more vulnerable than a simple area of dural exposure. Small, sessile meningoencephaloceles can be left alone if they are not involved with disease. Larger, broad-based meningoencephaloceles can be reduced and the tegmen defect repaired with cartilage, banked bone, split calvarial bone, hydroxyapatite discs, or synthetic commercially sold dura substitutes. Larger, pedunculated encephaloceles should be excised. The stalk can be fulgurated with bipolar cautery, and the lesion amputated. A CSF leak will often ensue and will need to be controlled with a multilayer repair, as described forthwith.

Spontaneous CSF leaks of the temporal bone are usually associated with intracranial hypertension, arachnoid granulations,[36] or previously undetected meningoencephaloceles with dural erosion (in children, spontaneous leaks are often associated with congenital anomalies of the inner ear). They can present with otorhinorrhea or be first discovered following myringotomy tube placement or an episode of meningitis.

CSF leaks should always be repaired. The presence of CSF leakage and the site of the leak may be difficult to verify preoperatively. When a leak is suspected, a fluid sample should be collected if possible. Testing for glucose (two thirds of the serum value) or chloride (higher than serum) content is suggestive but not definitive. Beta-2-transferrin assay is the most specific confirmatory test for CSF. It takes but a few drops of fluid to run the assay. It takes ~3 hours to complete, but this laboratory test is not routinely available at many laboratories. Shipping the aliquot of fluid to a designated laboratory requires a turnaround time of at least a few days. Beta-trace protein, a newer assay, may be just as sensitive, easier, and cheaper to run.

Once the presence of CSF is established, imaging studies are used to try to localize the site of the leak.[37] The single most useful study is a high-resolution CT scan. It may demonstrate

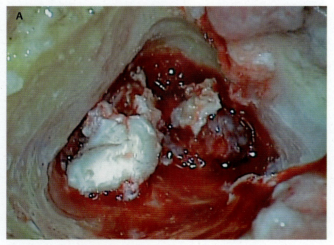
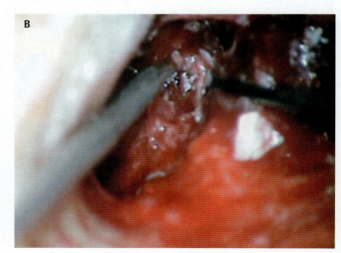

Fig. 6.22 **(A)** Cholesteatoma attached to bare dura on the tegmen, right ear. **(B)** After dural dissection.

the area of bony erosion of the tegmen or, less commonly, the posterior fossa dural plate; however, the bony defect may not correspond to the underlying dural defect that gave rise to the leak. Multiple tegmen defects and bilateral tegmen thinning are not uncommonly found and may introduce additional uncertainties. Magnetic resonance imaging (MRI) scanning in the coronal or sagittal plane will demonstrate an encephalocele but possibly not a meningocele. Radionuclide cisternography can definitively establish the presence of an active leak by showing pooling of intrathecally injected material in the mastoid. This imaging technique has low resolution and will not clearly demonstrate the location of the dural defect. The sensitivity of radionuclide testing can be enhanced by placing cottonoid pledgets in the nasal cavity and ear canal (if there is otorrhea) to look for radioactivity with a gamma counter; a positive test is diagnostic for CSF leakage but does not localize the site of the leak. CT cisternography with intrathecal contrast is the most precise method of localizing a leak, but it depends on a high rate of flow; slow or intermittent leaks will likely yield a negative study.

Ultimately, once the diagnosis of CSF leakage is made, surgical repair will be needed. At surgery, the site and size of the leak can be accurately determined, and a meningoencephalocele if present will usually be readily apparent. The use of intrathecal dyes or fluorescein is rarely necessary to visualize an occult leak in the mastoid. CSF leaks can be repaired from "above" (intracranially, using a middle cranial fossa approach), or from "below" (transmastoid).[38,39] The transmastoid approach is preferable for leaks that coexist with chronic middle ear disease when the defect is within the mastoid tegmen. Defects that are more anterior in the epitympanum, especially at or beyond the head of the malleus, are difficult to access without disarticulating the ossicular chain. A middle fossa approach may be necessary. The transcranial approach may also be more effective for controlling leaks that involve a larger area of dura, that involve multiple defects, or that recur after an unsuccessful transmastoid repair.[40]

The transcranial approach is performed through a middle cranial fossa (transtemporal) craniotomy. An extradural repair can be done by elevating the dura from the bony floor of the middle fossa and sliding a layer of fascia against the dural defect, then cartilage or split calvarial bone against the bony defect. An intradural repair is the most secure

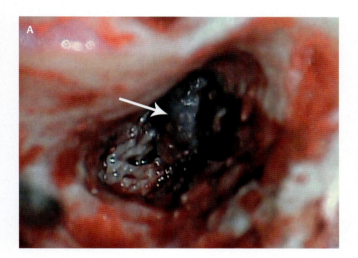

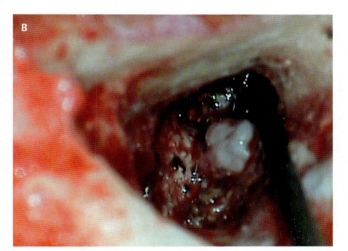

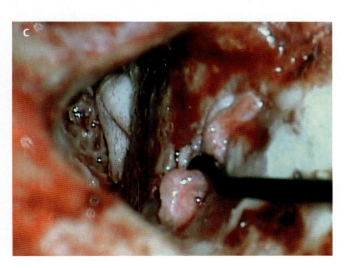

Fig. 6.23 Treatment of encephalocele arising through a tegmen defect, left ear. **(A)** Exposure of the encephalocele via canal wall up mastoidectomy. **(B)** Amputation of the stalk. **(C)** After dural repair using fascia plus cartilage graft.

method of repair and may be needed if the dura is attenuated. A dural incision is created along the lateral surface of the temporal lobe, then the brain is elevated and fascia, synthetic dura (Duragen Integra LifeSciences, Plainsboro, NJ), acellular dermis (AlloDerm, LifeCell Corp., Branchburg, NJ), or cadaveric pericardium placed between brain and dura. As the brain reexpands, the graft will be held firmly in place.

The transmastoid approach is performed by creating a canal wall up mastoidectomy and transmastoid atticotomy, exposing and skeletonizing the entire length of the tegmen (**Fig. 6.23A**). Once the leak is visualized, the surrounding bone is thinned with a diamond burr to maximize exposure. The tegmen can have an undulating contour so it should be skeletonized to a constant thickness. The healthy dura is carefully separated from the surrounding bone using a blunt elevator. If an encephalocele is present, it is either reduced or excised, depending on its size (**Fig. 6.23B**). A multilayer repair is undertaken by placing tissue against the dural defect (fascia, perichondrium, or AlloDerm can be used), then using stiffer material (cartilage, cortical bone, or banked bone) to repair the tegmen defect (**Fig. 6.23C**). The graft materials can be held in place by sandwiching them in the epidural space. As the intracranial contents expand they prevent the repair from migrating. Additional security can be gained by using fibrin glue over the repair and using an abdominal fat graft to fill the mastoid cavity.

When a CSF leak occurs in a canal wall down cavity, the mastoid cavity cannot be isolated from the ear canal as it can when the canal wall up is maintained. In this situation, the ear canal will usually have to be oversewn and the mastoid cavity obliterated with fat. The eustachian tube should also be sealed by packing muscle into the protympanum. If the area of leak is small, however, the area can sometimes be effectively sealed with hydroxyapatite bone cement (BoneSource, Stryker, Kalamazoo, MI; or Norian, Synthes, West Chester, PA). The bone cement should be covered with soft tissue, such as a skin flap or Palva flap, because it will become desiccated and behave as a foreign body if left exposed to the outside. This material should not be used in an infected cavity.

A case example is provided. A 45-year-old man with a history of bilateral cholesteatomas had undergone bilateral, staged, canal wall down mastoidectomies. The left ear, the better-hearing ear, developed decreasing hearing, and a soft tissue mass was found partially covering the eardrum and emerging from posterosuperiorly in the mastoid cavity. The mass was soft to palpation and did not contain any squamous elements. CT scan revealed a small breach in the tegmen mastoideum. The patient was brought to the operating room for

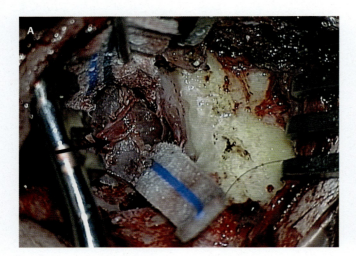

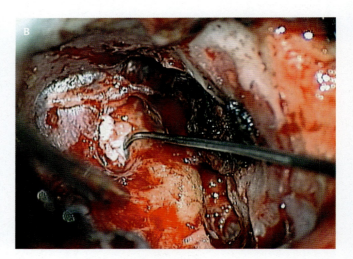

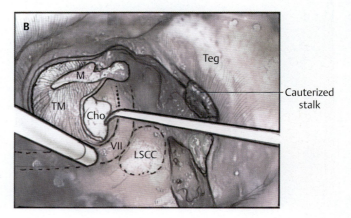

Fig. 6.24 Encephalocele (*arrow*) occurring in a canal wall down cavity, left ear. **(A)** Encephalocele dissected and isolated with cottonoids. **(B)** After multilayer dural repair with fascia and conchal cartilage.

surgical treatment with a preoperative differential diagnosis of encephalocele, residual cholesteatoma, or inflammatory cyst. At surgery, a large encephalocele was confirmed. The lesion was dissected from its mucosal attachments, and the neck was isolated (**Fig. 6.24A**). The neck was fulgurated with bipolar electrocautery, and the mass was excised. A small CSF leak developed intraoperatively. The bony tegmen was thinned with a diamond drill. The dural edges were bluntly elevated from the surrounding bone. A multilayer repair was performed using a temporalis fascia graft in the epidural space, and bone cement (Norian, Stryker) to repair the tegmen (**Fig. 6.24B**). A conchomeatal skin flap was developed to cover the bone cement. The CSF leak did not recur, but the skin flap retracted, and the bone cement became exposed and desiccated, with inflamed granulation tissue around its edges. Nine months later, with the inflammation controlled and the cavity perfectly dry, the meatoplasty was revised, drilling the bone cement down to a thin eggshell, and turning a thicker Palvatype (fibromuscular) flap over it. The cavity has remained dry with no evidence of recurrent cholesteatoma. The patient is able to wear a hearing aid effectively.

In certain instances, the leak will not be adequately controlled via a transmastoid approach, and a combined intra- and extracranial route will be needed. Some have advocated performing a "minicraniotomy," performing a mastoidectomy initially, then creating a narrow bony aperture through the squamosa through which the dura can be elevated off the bony floor of the middle fossa and an extradural repair performed.

◆ Conclusion

Cholesteatoma can be an aggressive disease that finds its way into places within the middle ear and mastoid that can be difficult to dissect and remove. The oval window, the sinus tympani, the exposed facial nerve, the fenestrated lateral semicircular canal, the petrous apex, and exposed or dehiscent dura are all dangerous places that can become involved with disease. The need for complete disease removal may create situations that can jeopardize inner ear and facial nerve function. These situations demand clear judgment, honed surgical skills, and experience to achieve successful surgical outcomes.

References

1. Jackler RK. The surgical anatomy of cholesteatoma. Otolaryngol Clin North Am 1989;22(5):883–896
2. Savić D, Djerić D. Cholesteatoma in the oval window niche. Eur Arch Otorhinolaryngol 1990;247(2):81–83
3. Hüttenbrink KB. Manipulating the mobile stapes during tympanoplasty: the risk of stapedial luxation. Laryngoscope 1993;103(6):668–672
4. Jahrsdoerfer RA, Johns ME, Cantrell RW. Labyrinthine trauma during ear surgery. Laryngoscope 1978;88(10):1589–1595
5. Smyth GD, Gormley PK. Preservation of cochlear function in the surgery of cholesteatomatous labyrinthine fistulas and oval window tympanosclerosis. Otolaryngol Head Neck Surg 1987;96(2):111–118
6. Sudhoff H, Tos M. Pathogenesis of sinus cholesteatoma. Eur Arch Otorhinolaryngol 2007;264(10):1137–1143
7. Holt JJ. Posterior sinus of the middle ear. Ann Otol Rhinol Laryngol 2007;116(6):457–461
8. Marchioni D, Alicandri-Ciufelli M, Grammatica A, Mattioli F, Presutti L. Pyramidal eminence and subpyramidal space: an endoscopic anatomical study. Laryngoscope 2010;120(3):557–564
9. Lau T, Tos M. Treatment of sinus cholesteatoma: long-term results and recurrence rate. Arch Otolaryngol Head Neck Surg 1988;114(12):1428–1434
10. Marchioni D, Mattioli F, Alicandri-Ciufelli M, Presutti L. Transcanal endoscopic approach to the sinus tympani: a clinical report. Otol Neurotol 2009;30(6):758–765
11. Pulec JL. Sinus tympani: retrofacial approach for the removal of cholesteatomas. Ear Nose Throat J 1996;75(2):77, 81–83, 86–88
12. Leonetti JP, Buckingham RA, Marzo SJ. Retraction cholesteatoma of the sinus tympani. Am J Otol 1996;17(6):823–826
13. Leonetti JP, Marzo SJ, Beauchamp MM, Jellish WS. Long-term results with operated sinus tympani retraction cholesteatoma. Otolaryngol Head Neck Surg 2006;135(1):152–154
14. Spielmann P, Mills RP. Surgical management of retraction pockets of the pars tensa with cartilage and perichondrial grafts. J Laryngol Otol 2006;120(9):725–729
15. Paparella MM, Jung TT. Experience with tympanoplasty for atelectatic ears. Laryngoscope 1981;91(9 Pt 1):1472–1477
16. Milewski C. Composite graft tympanoplasty in the treatment of ears with advanced middle ear pathology. Laryngoscope 1993;103(12):1352–1356
17. Avraham S, Luntz M, Sadé J. The influence of ventilating tubes on the surgical treatment of atelectatic ears. Eur Arch Otorhinolaryngol 1991;248(5):259–261
18. Elsheikh MN, Elsherief HS, Elsherief SG. Cartilage tympanoplasty for management of tympanic membrane atelectasis: is ventilatory tube necessary? Otol Neurotol 2006;27(6):859–864
19. Bayazit YA, Ozer E, Kanlikama M. Gross dehiscence of the bone covering the facial nerve in the light of otological surgery. J Laryngol Otol 2002;116(10):800–803
20. Moody MW, Lambert PR. Incidence of dehiscence of the facial nerve in 416 cases of cholesteatoma. Otol Neurotol 2007;28(3):400–404
21. Lin JC, Ho KY, Kuo WR, Wang LF, Chai CY, Tsai SM. Incidence of dehiscence of the facial nerve at surgery for middle ear cholesteatoma. Otolaryngol Head Neck Surg 2004;131(4):452–456
22. Selesnick SH, Lynn-Macrae AG. The incidence of facial nerve dehiscence at surgery for cholesteatoma. Otol Neurotol 2001;22(2):129–132
23. Parisier SC, Edelstein DR, Han JC, Weiss MH. Management of labyrinthine fistulas caused by cholesteatoma. Otolaryngol Head Neck Surg 1991;104(1):110–115
24. Copeland BJ, Buchman CA. Management of labyrinthine fistulae in chronic ear surgery. Am J Otolaryngol 2003;24(1):51–60
25. Vartiainen E. What is the best method of treatment for labyrinthine fistulae caused by cholesteatoma? Clin Otolaryngol Allied Sci 1992;17(3):258–260
26. Ostri B, Bak-Pedersen K. Surgical management of labyrinthine fistulae in chronic otitis media with cholesteatoma by a one-stage closed technique. ORL J Otorhinolaryngol Relat Spec 1989;51(5):295–299
27. Smouha EE, Namdar I, Michaelides EM. Partial labyrinthectomy with hearing preservation: an experimental study in guinea pigs. Otolaryngol Head Neck Surg 1996;114(6):777–784
28. Parnes LS, McClure JA. Effect on brainstem auditory evoked responses of posterior semicircular canal occlusion in guinea pigs. J Otolaryngol 1985;14(3):145–150
29. Vanden Abeele D, Offeciers FE. Management of labyrinthine fistulas in cholesteatoma. Acta Otorhinolaryngol Belg 1993;47(3):311–321
30. Kobayashi T, Shiga N, Hozawa K, Hashimoto S, Takasaka T. Effect on cochlear potentials of lateral semicircular canal destruction. Arch Otolaryngol Head Neck Surg 1991;117(11):1292–1295
31. Hakuba N, Hato N, Shinomori Y, Sato H, Gyo K. Labyrinthine fistula as a late complication of middle ear surgery using the canal wall down technique. Otol Neurotol 2002;23(6):832–835
32. Grayeli AB, Mosnier I, El Garem H, Bouccara D, Sterkers O. Extensive intratemporal cholesteatoma: surgical strategy. Am J Otol 2000;21(6):774–781
33. Moffat D, Jones S, Smith W. Petrous temporal bone cholesteatoma: a new classification and long-term surgical outcomes. Skull Base 2008;18(2):107–115
34. Bartels LJ. Facial nerve and medially invasive petrous bone cholesteatomas. Ann Otol Rhinol Laryngol 1991;100(4 Pt 1):308–316

35. Magliulo G, Terranova G, Sepe C, Cordeschi S, Cristofar P. Petrous bone cholesteatoma and facial paralysis. Clin Otolaryngol Allied Sci 1998;23(3):253–258

36. Gacek RR, Gacek MR, Tart R. Adult spontaneous cerebrospinal fluid otorrhea: diagnosis and management. Am J Otol 1999;20(6):770–776

37. Brown NE, Grundfast KM, Jabre A, Megerian CA, O'Malley BW Jr, Rosenberg SI. Diagnosis and management of spontaneous cerebrospinal fluid-middle ear effusion and otorrhea. Laryngoscope 2004;114(5):800–805

38. Sanna M, Fois P, Russo A, Falcioni M. Management of meningoencephalic herniation of the temporal bone: personal experience and literature review. Laryngoscope 2009;119(8):1579–1585

39. Wootten CT, Kaylie DM, Warren FM, Jackson CG. Management of brain herniation and cerebrospinal fluid leak in revision chronic ear surgery. Laryngoscope 2005;115(7):1256–1261

40. Pelosi S, Bederson JB, Smouha EE. Cerebrospinal fluid leaks of temporal bone origin: selection of surgical approach. Skull Base Surg 2010;20:253–259

7

Situations That Arise at Surgery: Hearing Issues

This chapter and the previous one address the unique situations that arise during cholesteatoma surgery. The prior chapter dealt with anatomical factors that confront surgeons. The current chapter deals with issues related to hearing. The preservation or restoration of hearing function is the second key goal of cholesteatoma surgery, and this is generally subservient to the complete removal (or exteriorization) of the disease. However, there are certain instances in which the hearing status will be an important issue in surgical timing and surgical decision making. These clinical instances are addressed in this chapter, and include the intact ossicular chain, cholesteatoma in the better-hearing ear, bilateral cholesteatoma, and cholesteatoma developing in an only hearing ear.

◆ Intact Ossicular Chain

Occasionally, the surgeon encounters an intact ossicular chain in the presence of cholesteatoma. It is tempting in these cases to try to maintain ossicular continuity in the interest of hearing preservation, but the surgical management should never compromise the complete removal of the disease. Good hearing outcomes can usually be expected even when the ossicular chain has to be reconstructed, and especially when the stapes superstructure can be preserved. On the other hand, leaving residual disease will eventually require additional surgery and lead to erosion of the ossicles, making long-term hearing preservation unlikely. When abundant inflammation is found at surgery, a normal hearing outcome is unlikely, even if the ossicular chain is preserved.

The preoperative hearing level does not correlate with the location and size of the cholesteatoma. Normal preoperative hearing is occasionally seen in cases with ossicular erosion because the cholesteatoma itself may conduct sound efficiently. In these cases, patients may be disappointed if they have postoperative hearing loss despite an otherwise good surgical outcome (**Fig. 7.1**). Conversely, preoperative hearing loss can occur in the presence of an intact ossicular chain because the cholesteatoma or associated inflammation impedes

the conduction of sound. Preserving the ossicular chain does not routinely lead to normal hearing in these cases.[1,2]

When an intact ossicular chain is found in the presence of normal preoperative hearing, the desire to maintain good hearing may conflict with the need to remove all the disease. Often the cholesteatoma can be removed without interrupting the ossicular chain, but this does not always result in normal postoperative hearing. In our series of cholesteatomas in normal-hearing ears, 72% had an intact ossicular chain, and ossicular continuity could be maintained in three fourths of these cases. Seventy-eight percent of patients with intact

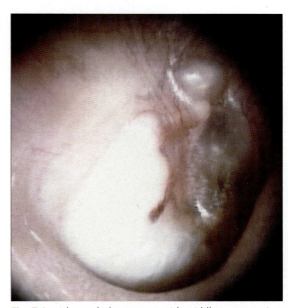

Fig. 7.1 A large cholesteatoma with middle ear extension and normal preoperative audiogram. The disease was removed completely via canal wall up mastoidectomy with preservation of an intact ossicular chain. Despite this, the patient developed a maximal conductive hearing loss. Second-stage surgery revealed no residual disease, but there was fibrosis of the ossicular chain, which precluded ossicular reconstruction.

ossicular chains achieved hearing preservation to within 7 dB at the initial audiogram, but this decreased to 61% long term.[1] In contrast, hearing preservation after ossicular reconstruction was 88% short term and 75% maintained long-term good outcomes. Reasons for long-term hearing decline include fibrosis, retraction, and disease recurrence.

An intact ossicular chain is often encountered in cases of congenital cholesteatomas, acquired cholesteatomas confined to the middle ear, or attic cholesteatomas limited to the Prussak space. Congenital cholesteatomas, if they are detected early, can usually be removed without disrupting the integrity of the eardrum or ossicular chain, and a normal hearing result can be maintained (see Chapter 9). Middle ear cholesteatomas can be associated with an intact ossicular chain if they are small and attached to the tympanic membrane or if they grow posteriorly and avoid the incus and stapes. In these cases, surgery can be done with ossicular preservation, but re-retraction can compromise the long-term hearing. Attic cholesteatoma confined to the Prussak space can often be removed with ossicular preservation.

Larger epitympanic cholesteatomas can also be handled this way if they spread posteriorly along the plane lateral to the incus (**Fig. 7.2A–D**). If disease extends more superiorly into the epitympanum but remains lateral to the incus and malleus, a Bondy mastoidectomy can be performed and the integrity of the ossicular chain preserved. Posterior epitympanic cholesteatoma usually envelops the incus, necessitating removal of the incus. Preserving the incus should be done very selectively in these instances because of the higher likelihood of residual disease. The endoscope may be helpful in assessing the completeness of cholesteatoma removal in these cases.[3]

◆ Cholesteatoma in the Better-Hearing Ear

Cholesteatoma usually occurs unilaterally and a less-than-perfect hearing outcome can be accepted when one good ear remains. However, when there is hearing loss in the opposite

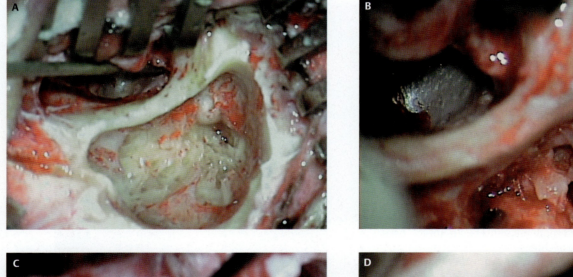

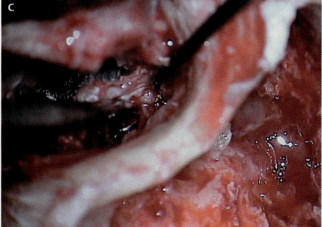
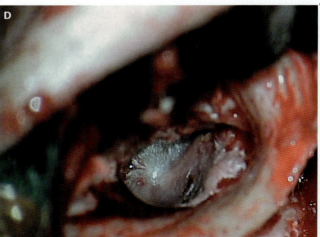

Fig. 7.2 **(A)** A lateral epitympanic space cholesteatoma of the left ear extending to the antrum, with an intact ossicular chain. **(B)** The sac was opened, and its contents were decompressed and delivered. **(C)** The remaining matrix was then dissected away from the lateral surface of the incus. The cholesteatoma was completely removed while preserving an intact ossicular chain. **(D)** The scutum was repaired with a cartilage graft, and the tympanomeatal flap was redraped over this.

ear, either from cholesteatoma or from an unrelated cause, hearing preservation is more crucial. The choice of surgical approach, and, indeed, the decision to operate at all, may be critical to the outcome.

Cholesteatoma occurs bilaterally in at least 8% of cases.[4] The majority of cases present simultaneously, but some will present sequentially.[5] When cholesteatoma affects both ears, patients will be subjected to multiple surgical operations, and the hearing outcome may be poor.[5,6] Complete disease removal with the lowest possible chance of recurrence is therefore paramount, and a canal wall down or Bondy approach will achieve these goals in most cases when the disease begins in the attic. Hearing preservation has greater significance in bilateral than in unilateral cases, and in most instances performing a canal wall down procedure will not introduce a hearing penalty.[7] In cases of middle ear cholesteatoma, a tympanoplasty approach will be used, and primary ossicular reconstruction can be undertaken. Obtaining a dry, stable ear is an important goal when a hearing aid will be needed. A bone-anchored cochlear stimulator (BAHA

Cochlear Americas, Centennial, CO)[8] or even a cochlear implant may be considered in certain instances.

A few cases are presented that illustrate the decision-making process when cholesteatoma occurs in a better-hearing ear.

Bilateral Cholesteatoma Presenting Sequentially

A 38-year-old male patient complained of progressive hearing loss in the right ear without drainage. He had undergone cholesteatoma surgery in the left ear 8 years earlier, with a poor hearing outcome. Examination revealed a dry attic retraction with squamous debris on the right side, and a canal wall down mastoidectomy on the left side with a small, dry cavity. Audiometry revealed bilateral conductive hearing loss, 35 dB on the right and 50 dB on the left. Computed tomography (CT) revealed a poorly developed mastoid on the right side with soft tissue density in the attic and antrum, enveloping the ossicles (**Fig. 7.3A**).

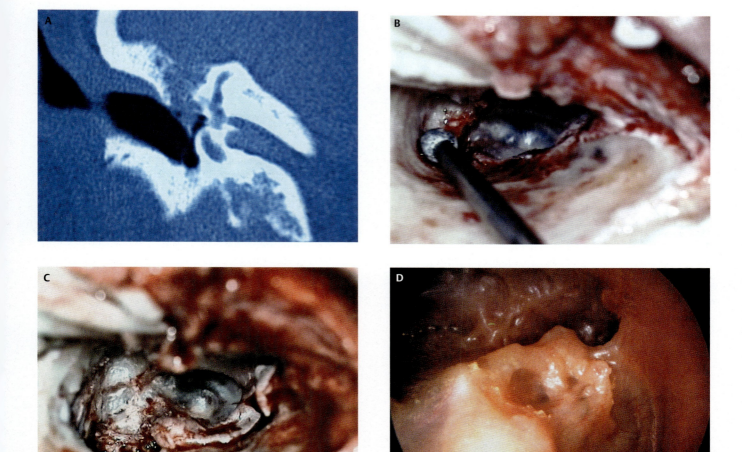

Fig. 7.3 **(A)** Computed tomographic scan showing an attic cholesteatoma in the better-hearing ear. **(B)** Bondy operation, right ear. Transcanal atticotomy is performed to exteriorize disease. **(C)** The atticotomy is enlarged back to the antrum by following the tegmen posteriorly, exteriorizing the cholesteatoma sac. As drilling progresses, a round, beveled cavity is created. **(D)** Postoperative appearance of Bondy mastoidectomy–intact tympanic membrane, exteriorized attic, and antrum.

A Bondy operation (inside-out canal wall down mastoidectomy) is the ideal operation in this situation. The decision to operate is not optional, and the need to preserve hearing is paramount. The goal is to remove the cholesteatoma and preserve the ossicular chain while avoiding the middle ear space entirely if possible.

The procedure is done through a postauricular approach. Working through the ear canal with a diamond burr, the attic is opened first to identify the tegmen tympani laterally near the outer cortex. The tegmen is then followed medially toward the epitympanum. The scutum is thinned down to an eggshell and then removed with a curette to avoid vibrational trauma from the drill to the ossicles. The atticotomy is enlarged back to the antrum, again by following the tegmen posteriorly (**Fig. 7.3B,C**). The goal is to completely exteriorize the cholesteatoma sac. As drilling progresses, a round, beveled cavity is created. In a sclerotic ear, the surgeon can use a diamond burr to contour the bone to create a cavity of manageable shape and size. This requires beveling or saucerizing the cortical bony edges and lowering the facial ridge to the level of the fibrous annulus. It is possible to do this without separating the annulus or entering the middle ear. In sclerotic mastoids, the mastoid tip is usually not developed and does not need to be opened.

The resulting surgical exposure allows complete removal of the disease under direct vision. This can be done without removing the incus or disrupting the incudostapedial joint, if the disease has not involved these structures. Closure of the cavity is done by draping the conchomeatal flap along the sinodural angle; fascial grafting of the medial attic wall is optional. The postoperative appearance is a compact cavity with an intact tympanic membrane (TM), and the attic is exteriorized (**Fig. 7.3D**). This has a low chance of recurrence or postoperative drainage. The hearing results are generally very good. The compact cavity permits the use of a hearing aid without fear of drainage or maceration.

The Bondy operation is not suitable for cases of middle ear cholesteatoma. An illustrative example is a young man who had a previous canal wall down mastoidectomy for large cholesteatoma in the right ear that resulted in a dry cavity, but with a large conductive hearing loss. Second-stage ossicular reconstruction was unsuccessful because of middle ear fibrosis. The patient returned 1 year later with hearing loss and a single episode of drainage from the opposite ear.

Examination revealed a cholesteatoma sac in the left middle ear (**Fig. 7.4A**). The disease was removed via transmeatal approach, raising a tympanomeatal flap and performing a limited atticotomy until sufficient exposure was gained. The scutum was reconstructed with tragal cartilage, and the hearing remained normal. After 5 years, the patient developed a recurrence beneath the cartilage graft. This was reexcised via a transmeatal approach. **Figure 7.4B** shows the middle ear disease traveling lateral to the incus to the Prussak space; this was removed completely, with mirror confirmation (**Fig. 7.4C**) and the scutum again closed with tragal cartilage. The patient maintained normal hearing after the revision procedure after 8 more years of follow-up.

Bilateral Cholesteatoma Presenting Simultaneously

Simultaneous bilateral cholesteatoma presents a challenge. Generally one ear will be more symptomatic, with active drainage and worse hearing, and this ear should be operated on first. The less symptomatic ear can be dealt with in a staged fashion, once the first ear heals and is stable. If the second side is the better-hearing ear, it may be tempting to defer surgery as long as possible, or the patient may not wish to have the second operation, but this may be just delaying the inevitable. If the cholesteatoma grows or becomes infected it may compromise the hearing in the better ear and make the ossicular reconstruction more difficult. Some case examples follow.

A 65-year-old man presented with refractory bilateral chronic ear drainage for 3 years. The right ear had copious purulent drainage and squamous material emerging from the attic; the left ear had a small attic retraction with moderate drainage. CT showed bilateral compact mastoids with soft tissue densities and erosion of the lateral semicircular canal on the right. Audiometry showed severe mixed hearing loss in the right ear and moderately severe loss on the left.

He underwent right radical mastoidectomy first, because this was the more problematic and poorer-hearing ear, with the plan of performing staged surgery on the left ear at a later date. At surgery, an infected cholesteatoma was removed, and a lateral semicircular canal fistula was identified, unroofed, and sealed with periosteum. Cultures yielded *Pseudomonas*. Postoperatively he developed an anacoustic ear and vertigo

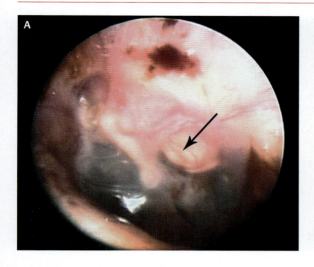

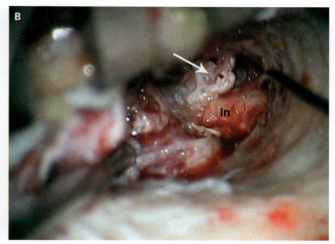

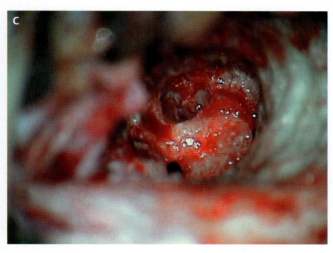

Fig. 7.4 (A) Recurrent cholesteatoma, right ear (*arrow*). This is an attic cholesteatoma beginning in the pars flaccida and extending to the middle ear, in the better-hearing ear. **(B)** A transmeatal approach was used. The disease (*arrow*) filled the Prussak space and was dissected off the lateral surface of the incus (In) and malleus. It was excised, maintaining an intact ossicular chain. **(C)** An intact ossicular chain was preserved, and the postoperative audiogram showed only a mild conductive loss.

that resolved slowly despite treatment with intravenous (IV) antibiotics. Four months later, he developed right facial paralysis. He was hospitalized for presumed *Pseudomonas* osteitis and given IV imipenem. The facial paralysis, imbalance, and otorrhea resolved completely, but profound sensorineural hearing loss remained.

The left ear continued to drain intermittently, even during IV antibiotic therapy. *Pseudomonas* was also confirmed by culture. It was decided that surgical treatment could no longer be avoided. Because this was now an only hearing ear, a modified radical mastoidectomy was performed through an

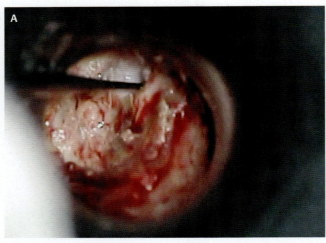
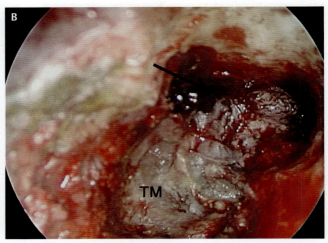

Fig. 7.5 **(A)** Attic cholesteatoma in only hearing ear, right side, before (with pick in attic defect), and **(B)** after transmeatal excision with preservation of middle ear and tympanic membrane (TM). The atticoantrotomy is visible (*arrow*).

endaural approach (**Fig. 7.5A,B**). The goal was to do the least invasive operation that would control the disease, minimize the risk of further hearing loss, and minimize the need for postoperative packing. The ear healed well, with an intact tympanic membrane and an open attic-antral cavity. Because he received limited benefit from a hearing aid, a bone-anchored cochlear stimulator (BAHA, Cochlear Americas, Centennial, CO) was later implanted on the right side. The patient was very happy with the hearing that this afforded him, and both ears have remained dry and stable.

Cholesteatoma Developing in an Only Hearing Ear

A 48-year-old man presented with sudden sensorineural hearing loss in the right ear and failed to recover any hearing despite treatment with oral steroids, antivirals, and diuretics. His final hearing level was 80 dB PTA, with poor speech discrimination, hyperacusis, and distorted hearing with amplification.

He had a history of chronic otitis media in his left ear and had a posterior pars tensa retraction pocket with a natural myringostapediopexy. His hearing was normal on the left side. He had intermittent otorrhea from the left ear that would cause a decline in hearing. The problem cleared quickly after the use of antibiotic drops. Over time, the episodes of otorrhea increased in frequency, and the hearing loss became more persistent. Endoscopic exam of the ear revealed a deep retraction pocket in the attic in addition to the middle ear (**Fig. 7.6**). There was pus but no squamous debris present. CT revealed focal thickening of the tympanic membrane in the middle ear and in the attic.

The patient developed a retraction pocket cholesteatoma in his better-hearing ear. The opposite ear was not aidable.

The remaining options include continued conservative management or surgical treatment. He was advised to have surgery because of the progressive nature of the disease and because of the persistence of infection. He delayed his decision to have surgery for fear of losing more hearing.

In this case, a Bondy operation would take care of the disease in the attic but not the middle ear. A cartilage tympanoplasty is desirable for the posterior pars tensa retraction, but it would be difficult to perform without separating the myringostapediopexy and risking postoperative hearing loss. The patient has chosen to temporize and has avoided further episodes of otorrhea by exercising strict dry ear precautions.

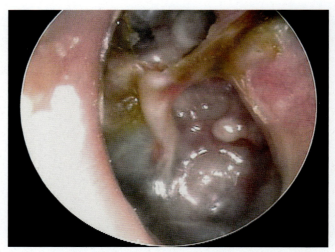

Fig. 7.6 Cholesteatoma in the better-hearing ear, right side. The attic retraction has progressively enlarged. The patient has intermittent drainage and has tried to avoid surgery.

There is no guarantee that he will develop disease progression that will make surgery unavoidable in the future.

◆ Conclusion

Hearing is an important issue in cholesteatoma surgery and one that affects surgical decision making. When an intact ossicular chain is encountered, it can sometimes be preserved, but complete removal of the disease must take precedence over preserving ossicular continuity. When cholesteatoma occurs in the better-hearing ear or in an only hearing ear, the surgical strategy must take hearing outcome into account, and a Bondy procedure is favored when appropriate. In cases of bilateral cholesteatoma, the more symptomatic ear is operated on first, again considering the eventual hearing outcome when planning the surgical strategy.

References

1. Smouha EE, Javidfar J. Cholesteatoma in the normal hearing ear. Laryngoscope 2007;117(5):854–858
2. Sakagami M, Seo T, Node M, Fukazawa K, Sone M, Mishiro Y. Cholesteatoma otitis media with intact ossicular chain. Auris Nasus Larynx 1999;26(2):147–151
3. Tarabichi M. Endoscopic management of limited attic cholesteatoma. Laryngoscope 2004;114(7):1157–1162
4. Edelstein DR, Parisier SC. Surgical techniques and recidivism in cholesteatoma. Otolaryngol Clin North Am 1989;22(5):1029–1040
5. Lin V, Daniel S, James A, Friedberg J. Bilateral cholesteatomas: the hospital for sick children experience. J Otolaryngol 2004;33(3):145–150
6. Vartiainen E. Fate of patients with bilateral cholesteatoma. Am J Otolaryngol 1993;14(1):49–52
7. Murphy TP, Wallis DL. Hearing results in pediatric patients after canal-wall-up and canal-wall-down mastoid surgery. Otolaryngol Head Neck Surg 1998;119(5):439–443
8. Wazen JJ, Spitzer J, Ghossaini SN, Kacker A, Zschommler A. Results of the bone-anchored hearing aid in unilateral hearing loss. Laryngoscope 2001;111(6):955–958

8

Controversies in Cholesteatoma Surgery

There are a few areas in cholesteatoma management that remain controversial, where experienced surgeons continue to hold fundamental differences of opinion about treatment options. The canal wall up versus canal wall down debate is chief among these and has endured despite decades of accumulated clinical evidence and shifting viewpoints. The question of second-stage (or "second-look") surgery has also persisted, and yet uncertainty remains about what to do if recurrent disease is found. Facial nerve monitoring has found a place in the surgical management of cholesteatoma and chronic ear disease, but despite its widespread use, there continues to be disagreement about its value and about its proper method of implementation. Endoscopes, which have gained broad acceptance in other areas of otolaryngology and skull base surgery, have not replaced the microscope in the treatment of ear disease and yet have found some suitable applications in the management of cholesteatoma and in the detection of recurrence. The adequacy of follow-up is a factor that continues to be vital in controlling this disease, because of the persistently high rate of recurrence.

These areas of controversy are discussed in detail here.

◆ Canal Wall Up versus Canal Wall Down

The ideal treatment for cholesteatoma is a single-stage operation with a very low recurrence rate and no need for bowl maintenance. Such a procedure still does not exist, however, and so debate continues about the relative merits of canal wall up (CWU) and canal wall down (CWD) procedures. The controversy between CWU versus CWD surgery reached its pinnacle in the 1960s and '70s, when vocal and colorful advocates of each position argued, with a certain amount of zealotry, for one approach at the exclusion of the other. As with most trends in medicine, a more balanced view took hold over time, with the recognition that each approach was appropriate in certain situations.

The CWD technique (also called open cavity or modified radical mastoidectomy) has a low rate of residual disease that can be detected and treated in the office, and a (theoretically) zero rate of recurrent disease, albeit at the expense of creating a mastoid cavity. CWD therefore results in a "safe" ear. Published studies have shown CWD to have a lower recurrence rate than CWU, with a rate varying from 0% to less than 10% in studies with at least 10 years follow-up. However, the cavity is an alteration of the normal anatomy, a reservoir for accumulation of cerumen and epithelial debris, and a potential area for mucositis and persistent postoperative drainage. Because of the need for periodic cleaning and water precautions, the CWD procedure carries a penalty, especially for children.

CWU avoids the problems of an open cavity, but at the cost of a higher rate of recurrent/residual disease. The CWU technique, also called closed cavity, combined approach, and intact canal wall, preserves the posterior bony canal wall and results in a normal ear canal without a cavity. The advantages of CWU are preservation of normal anatomy, more rapid healing, and (as is often claimed), better hearing. The disadvantage of CWU is the possibility of residual cholesteatoma (disease left behind by the surgeon) behind an intact wall, and the risk of recurrence (re-formation of cholesteatoma from a new retraction pocket), usually in the attic beneath the bony scutum. The incidence of residual disease has led many advocates of CWU to recommend a second-stage operation, usually 6 to 18 months after the initial operation, to examine for and treat such a possibility.

Except in the eyes of the most dogmatic surgeons, each technique has a proper role in the management of cholesteatoma. The determining factors are the size of the mastoid, the extent of the disease, the presence of a complication (such as labyrinthine fistula), and the reliability of the patient for follow-up. Patients with sclerotic mastoids can be safely and easily treated with CWD, which results in a compact cavity with little risk of recurrence or postoperative drainage. Patients with large, extensively pneumatized mastoids are better treated with CWU when their disease permits, because

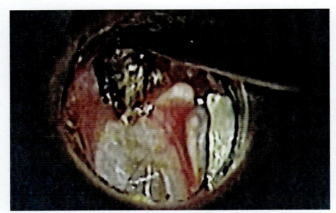

Fig. 8.1 Otomicroscopic view of right ear, showing probing of attic cholesteatoma.

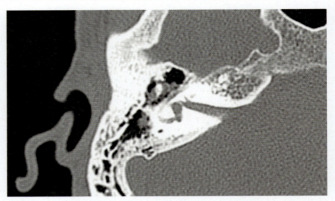

Fig. 8.2 Computed tomographic scan of the same patient, showing an attic-antral cholesteatoma, enveloping ossicles.

postoperative cavity maintenance could be problematic. Extensive cholesteatomas are better treated with CWD because of their greater likelihood for recurrence; small, well-localized cholesteatomas can be adequately managed with CWU. Complications are usually better managed by CWD because of the overriding need to create a safe ear. Recurrences too are usually managed with CWD. Unreliable or migratory patients are better treated with CWD.

Preoperative computed tomographic (CT) scanning is helpful for surgical planning. CT reveals the size of the mastoid, the extent of the disease, and the presence of complications, including labyrinthine fistula, facial nerve or tegmen or sigmoid sinus dehiscence, or disease invasion into difficult areas. Although CT is not mandatory, in most cases it is nice to have.

In many, if not most, cases, the decision to leave the canal wall or take the canal wall down can be made at surgery. Patients are usually consented (generically) for tympanomastoidectomy and are told that the procedure may result in a cavity and may require a second operation, depending on the surgical findings. In this "flexible" or "eclectic" approach, the mastoid is approached though a postauricular incision, and a CWU mastoidectomy is performed first. Once the extent of the disease and the difficulty of dissection are determined, the surgeon can decide whether or not to take the canal wall down.

In practice, the two areas that might be most problematic for a CWU approach are the sinus tympani and the anterior epitympanic space. The following case illustrates this approach in practice. A 40-year-old woman complained of intermittent drainage and hearing loss in her right ear. Examination revealed a dry crust over the pars flaccida; gentle debridement revealed a deep retraction pocket with squamous debris and scutum erosion (**Fig. 8.1**). An audiogram revealed a 40 dB conductive hearing loss. CT revealed soft tissue in the attic and antrum (**Fig. 8.2**).

At surgery, the lesion was first explored through the meatus. By probing the attic retraction pocket, it was seen that the sac extended back to the epitympanum. A CWU mastoidectomy was created with transmastoid atticotomy and facial recess (**Fig. 8.3**). The sac was incised in the antrum, its contents were evacuated, and it was delivered forward toward the middle ear. The incus was removed, and the malleus head was cut with a nipper. There was found to be more extensive involvement than indicated by the CT, with disease extending toward the anterior epitympanic space (**Fig. 8.4**).

At this juncture, the surgeon has to decide whether the cholesteatoma can be completely removed via a CWU approach, or whether the canal wall should be taken down. In this case, exposure of the anterior epitympanic space was compromised by a low-lying tegmen—the posterior bony canal wall could not be thinned any further without

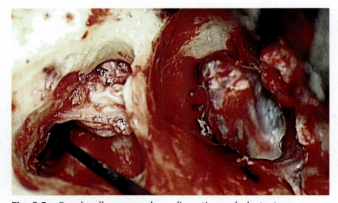

Fig. 8.3 Canal wall up procedure, dissecting a cholesteatoma sac from the mastoid antrum.

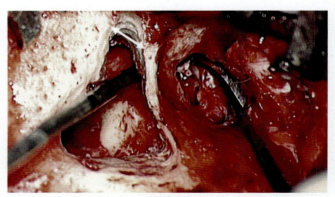

Fig. 8.4 Transmastoid atticotomy, with disease remaining in the attic. Vertical height of the tegmen (*arrows*) limits the view of the anterior epitympanum.

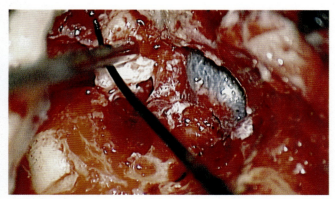

Fig. 8.5 After conversion to canal wall down, there is a clear view of residual disease in the attic.

perforating it, so it was decided to take the canal wall down (**Fig. 8.5**) (another option in this case would be a transcanal atticotomy, removing the scutum to gain anterior exposure, and reconstructing it later with cartilage).

Choosing between CWU or CWD is often not a black and white decision, as this case illustrates. If CWU is selected, the patient may need a second-stage (second-look) operation to search for residual disease, or may risk developing a recurrent cholesteatoma through the scutum graft. If CWD is performed, the risk of recurrence will be lower but a cavity will result. Several techniques of canal wall reconstruction have been proposed to mitigate the cavity factor.

Canal Wall Reconstruction

Reconstruction of the canal wall in mastoid surgery is not a new concept. It may have been introduced by Mosher[1] and was later utilized by Wullstein[2] and others. Different techniques and materials have since been used in an effort to decrease cavity size and prevent recurrent disease. The musculocutaneous flap described by Silvola and Palva,[3] using temporalis muscle and fibrous tissue pedicled to the conchomeatal skin, is a widely popular means of reducing cavity size but often retracts and does not completely eliminate the mastoid bowl (the technique is described in Chapter 5). Bone pate, which is readily available in the surgical field, is commonly used for cavity obliteration, but the material may resorb or become infected. It might never completely solidify, or it may contain squamous elements that can lead to recurrence.[4]

Mercke[5] introduced a technique of mastoid reconstruction reimplanting the posterior canal wall and obliterating the cavity with bone chips. This technique resulted in no recurrent cholesteatoma and reduced rate of residual, dry ear, and intact tympanic membrane (TM), and it improved upon the results obtained with CWU and CWD. Gantz et al,[6] in 2005, published a series of 127 patients who underwent a similar procedure, with a recurrence rate of 1.5% at 4 years mean follow-up. This technique improved on the recurrence rate when compared with CWU, but wound infections were relatively common, requiring inpatient intravenous (IV) antibiotics. In addition, the procedure did not eliminate the need

for a second-look operation, and the ossicular chain was routinely sacrificed at the first operation, with ossicular reconstruction delayed until the second stage.

McElveen and Chung[7] introduced a "reversible canal wall down" technique, in which the bony canal wall is removed then refixated using bone cement. Although only five cases were described, the technique appears to provide good surgical exposure but results in a CWU-type cavity with the same potential for recurrence.

"Soft wall" reconstruction has also been attempted, first by Smith et al,[8] and later by Takahashi et al,[9] in which a portion of the posterior canal wall is removed for surgical exposure and later replaced by temporalis fascia and canal skin. Recurrence/residual rates were similar to those for CWD, but retraction of the canal skin into the mastoid bowl occurred in nearly 50% of cases. Dornhoffer[10] advocated reconstruction of the canal wall with cartilage from the cimbum concha, and reported an 18% recurrence rate and excellent hearing results with this technique. Although these results are quite acceptable, rigid techniques appear to yield a lower rate of recurrence.

Several foreign materials have been used to obliterate the mastoid cavity. Hydroxyapatite (HA) granules and implants have shown favorable results, but HA cement may have a high rate of infection.[11] HA canal wall implants failed 25% of cases, usually because of middle ear infection rather than recurrent cholesteatoma.[12] Ceravital, a bioactive ceramic glass, has also been successful, but its use is cautioned against in patients with immunologic disorders or diabetes.[13] Titanium implants have also been used to reconstruct the canal wall.[14] Hard materials such as these may eliminate the cavity problem but also may hinder the detection of the recurrent cholesteatoma. Because of the need for meticulous fitting and for vascularized soft tissue coverage, rigid implant materials have not gained widespread use, and concern remains over the potential for infection or extrusion.

We have used an alternative technique of reconstructed canal wall mastoidectomy in which the posterior canal wall is removed en bloc and then reused as a free bone graft to obliterate the sinodural angle (**Figs. 8.6, 8.7,** and **8.8**). The surgical exposure is the same as for CWD, so the chance of leaving disease behind is very low. The attic remains exteriorized, thereby preventing recurrent disease from forming in that location. No foreign material or bone pate is used; therefore there is no increased risk of infection and little risk of

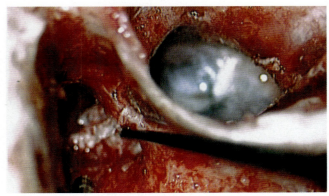

Fig. 8.6 Attic cholesteatoma, with a low-lying tegmen.

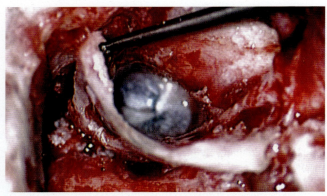

Fig. 8.7 The posterior bony canal wall is removed en bloc after opening the facial recess and drilling troughs superiorly at its attachment to the tegmen, and inferiorly at the mastoid tip.

reimplanting disease. The procedure still results in the creation of a cavity, but the size of the cavity is lessened, both by the reimplantation of cortical bone from the posterior canal, and by maintaining the mastoid tip. The bony reconstruction blocks the sinodural angle and results in a cavity no deeper than the lateral semicircular canal (**Fig. 8.8**). Using a conchomeatal flap in conjunction with the bony obliteration re-

sults in a round bowl with sloping edges, and a functionally small cavity with little surface area to collect debris.

Obliteration techniques carry the potential risk of burying residual disease, and so would not be advisable in cases of giant aggressive cholesteatoma, "cholesteatosis," or plunging disease.

◆ The Timing and Necessity of Second-Stage (Second-Look) Surgery for Cholesteatoma

Second-stage surgery is a decision that is made at the time of the initial operation. There are several reasons for choosing to perform a second stage:

1. Invasive cholesteatoma into the mucosa of the middle ear, anterior or posterior epitympanum, antrum, or mastoid
2. Cholesteatoma in a location such that the surgeon questions the success of total removal at the first stage
3. Previous failed surgery for tympanomastoid surgery with chronic otitis media and significant mucosal disease
4. Significant allergic or gastroesophageal reflux

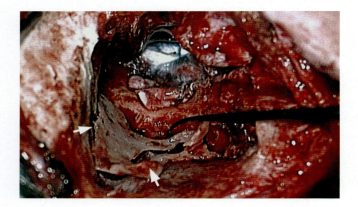

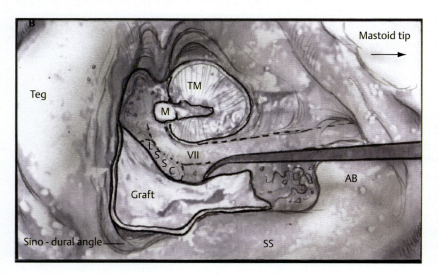

Fig. 8.8 Reconstructed canal wall. The bony implant is used to fill the sinodural angle (*arrows*), leaning it forward with its base against the facial ridge. The attic remains open.

5. Contracted middle ear space with an attempt to lateralize the middle ear cleft with a Silastic (Dow Corning, Midland, MI) implant (may include CWU or CWD procedures)

The main purpose of second-stage surgery is to search for the presence of residual disease after a CWU operation. The second purpose of second-stage surgery is to reconstruct the hearing mechanism in a staged fashion, at a time when the middle ear is stable and without disease.

The second-stage operation was originally recommended as a routine measure to detect residual disease by the proponents of CWU surgery. The main disadvantage of the CWU procedure is the possibility of recidivistic disease, which can either take the form of residual cholesteatoma (an epithelial remnant left in the mastoid cavity, anterior or posterior epitympanic space, or middle ear, separate from the tympanic membrane), or recurrent cholesteatoma (arising from a new tympanic membrane retraction). The former can grow silently behind an intact canal wall and tympanic membrane, and so a second-stage surgery is therefore recommended as a way to detect and treat the growth early, before it has had the opportunity to become destructive. The latter are clinically evident and can be detected without an additional surgical operation.

The further rationale for a staged second operation is to perform ossicular reconstruction in a stable middle ear. Cholesteatoma is destructive, and the ossicles are frequently eroded or separated by the disease. Primary ossicular reconstruction does not always meet with uniform success because of the presence of inflammation at the time of the original surgery, as well as the vagaries of healing. The tympanic membrane may become scarred, retracted, or adherent to the middle ear mucosa over time, and this may negatively influence the results of attempted ossicular repair. The odds of success may be improved if ossiculoplasty is undertaken at a later time, when there is no cholesteatoma present and the middle ear is not inflamed. In a stable middle ear, the height of the tympanic membrane relative to the stapes footplate will remain constant during healing, and so an ossicular prosthesis or sculpted incus can be sized and positioned accurately and predictably during surgery and will not be expected to shift or change.

The main objection to second-stage surgery is that it requires a separate trip to the operating room, subjecting the patient to additional anesthesia, surgical risk, and cost. It should be noted that many second-stage surgeries may be performed under IV sedation techniques markedly reducing risks of operation. Experience with local anesthesia techniques and IV sedation allows limited risk and immediate results of hearing improvement. Opponents of the second-stage approach will also argue that the second look will be negative in a significant proportion of cases, and that clinical follow-up alone is adequate because residual disease will make itself known in time. In some surgeons' hands, primary ossicular reconstruction yields good results in the majority of cases so that reconstruction need not be postponed to a later stage.

Certain issues remain unresolved about the role of second-stage surgery for cholesteatoma. First, there is disagreement about whether a second-stage operation should be *routinely*

performed after CWU operation, and whether for residual disease or for hearing or both. Although some surgeons still perform a planned second-stage after every case, many will do this selectively in cases where the completeness of excision was not certain (eg, in the sinus tympani, scutum, anterior or posterior epitympanic space, or mucosal invasion), or where the dissection was difficult because the disease was adherent or the anatomy did not allow unhindered exposure. The second stage also offers an opportunity to perform ossicular reconstruction in a "clean" field, as already discussed.

A second unresolved question is the optimal timing of the second operation. Most will perform the surgery as early as 6 months or as late as 2 years. Earlier surgery allows for residual disease to be dealt with when it is smaller and well circumscribed. Later surgery allows for maturation of scar tissue and a more stable middle ear space. For instance when the surgeon is trying to reconstruct and enlarge the middle ear cleft, waiting longer allows time for conformity of the middle ear space with the spacer Silastic sheeting enlarging this space. The timing remains a matter of individual preference.

A further unresolved question is how to deal with recurrence when it is found. This must be individualized by the situation found at surgery. The most conservative (but radical) approach would be to convert to a CWD mastoidectomy. This approach would virtually eliminate the possibility of further recurrence, but might result in a large, unwieldy cavity and would be overkill in the case of a small residual pearl. It is possible to leave the middle ear cleft by keeping the canal wall over the fallopian canal partially in place where the chorda tympani is located. On the other hand, maintaining an intact canal wall would be risky if extensive or invasive disease is discovered. In such a case, the surgeon may decide on performing a third stage with the suggestion that hearing improvement up to normalized hearing is potentially still possible. Many patients would not look forward to the prospect of a third operation, but in our experience, the surgeon–patient relationship and surgeon experience are key to this decision.

The technique of second-stage surgery presents certain options. The most formal method would consist of raising a tympanomeatal flap and reopening the mastoid through a postauricular incision. A more limited method would be to raise the tympanomeatal flap and use a mirror or endoscope to inspect the epitympanum or antrum. This technique might miss disease in the mastoid; however, some surgeons have used a small stab incision to pass a slim 2.7 or 4 mm endoscope into the mastoid. A limited procedure such as this can even be performed under local anesthesia. If extensive residual disease is found, the incision can be opened and a formal revision mastoidectomy performed.

Concerns remain about the yield of second-stage surgery and the adequacy of follow-up. In most studies, residual disease will be found in ~20 to 50% of second-look operations, meaning that the majority of operations will result in a negative exploration. This argues for a selective approach to second-look surgery and makes limited, endoscopically assisted surgery more attractive. Imaging techniques such as CT and magnetic resonance imaging (MRI) have been tried in an effort to avoid routine surgical exploration, but their predictive value is not perfect. CT cannot distinguish between one type of soft tissue and another, so postoperative fibrosis and residual disease might look the same. MRI likewise lacks specificity, although newer protocols such as diffusion-weighted imaging might improve on this. Issues of expense and patient discomfort persist with MRI, however.

Not all patients will agree to second surgery, and not all patients will return for regular follow-up, so some cases of residual disease will certainly be missed despite all efforts to be thorough. In a recent study from the New York Eye and Ear Infirmary (pers. comm.), the rate of follow-up after cholesteatoma surgery was around 50%, a rate that raises concern. It is important to realize that the doctor–patient relationship is crucial. Personally, in our preoperative education we talk to patients about their disease and that surgery is done in two stages to look for recurrent or residual cholesteatoma and optimize their hearing back toward normal limits.

◆ Facial Nerve Monitoring

The facial nerve is at risk during chronic ear surgery, and facial nerve injury remains a dreaded complication. The incidence of facial nerve paralysis during surgery is low, certainly less than 1% in experienced hands, but even so the threat of a facial nerve complication remains a sobering reality. Experienced surgeons recognize the fact that distorted anatomy, congenital anomalies, or extensive inflammatory disease can expose the facial nerve to unexpected surgical trauma even when every precaution is exercised.

It is therefore not surprising that the use of facial nerve monitoring has become commonplace during ear surgery. Nerve monitors have become seamless in their design and reliable in their performance, and have shown themselves to be helpful in difficult situations. Nevertheless, monitoring is not a substitute for an intimate knowledge of facial nerve anatomy or for meticulous surgical technique. Facial nerve monitoring should be seen as an adjunct, an extra layer of protection during surgery.

The purpose of the facial nerve stimulator/monitor is to help locate the nerve anatomically, to provide live feedback when dissecting on an exposed nerve, and to verify the functional integrity of the nerve by electrical stimulation. Facial nerve monitoring does not replace technical proficiency, anatomical knowledge, or the judgment that comes from surgical experience. The facial nerve monitor provides *contextual* information during surgery that must be interpreted within the situation at hand.

The principles of facial nerve monitoring have been outlined in detail in several sources.[15,16] A few devices are commercially available for monitoring the facial nerve during surgery. These devices contain two separate electric circuits, one to *stimulate* the nerve electrically, and the other to *monitor* the activity of the facial muscles.

The nerve stimulator allows the surgeon to apply a small electrical current to the nerve during surgery. This provides immediate information about the anatomical location and the functional integrity of the nerve. Electrical stimulation is delivered through a probe. Stimulator probes usually operate in a monopolar mode, dispersing current radially from the tip of the stimulator probe (bipolar probes, which emit current between two probe tips, are also available, but they are less often used because the current must be oriented parallel to the nerve).[17] Special surgical instruments also exist that can deliver an electric stimulus during dissection.[18] Stimulators are usually set to deliver a constant current, and the current level can be selected on the device (constant voltage devices also exist but can deliver excessive current if the tissue resistance is low). Typically, a current level of 1 to 2 mA (mA) will be needed to stimulate the facial nerve through an intact bony covering, whereas a very small current (0.1 mA) will stimulate a bare nerve. Stimulation will spread bidirectionally along the nerve. In the setting of facial nerve injury, the nerve will continue to stimulate distal to the site of the lesion for up to 3 days, even after complete transaction. Stimulation proximal to the site of the lesion will give information as to the degree of injury; brisk stimulation at a low current level implies functional continuity of the nerve, whereas a high stimulation threshold or complete absence of stimulation implies a severe conduction block or a transected nerve. Constant-current stimulation is susceptible to shunting, wherein the current is dissipated by any electrolytic fluid (blood, saline, CSF) in the surgical field; the field should be dried with a suction before attempting to stimulate the nerve.

The nerve monitor most commonly employs electromyography (EMG) to detect contraction of the facial muscles during surgery, although there are motion sensors ("strain gauge sensors") that have a higher threshold for detecting a response. The monitor produces an audible signal (as well as a visual oscilloscopic tracing) in response to facial muscle contraction. The audible signal provides live feedback to the surgeon during the dissection. The facial nerve monitor typically allows for recording from two or more channels during

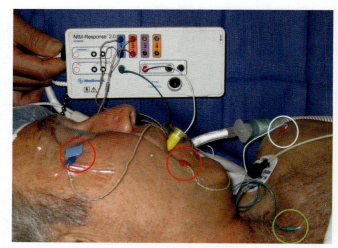

Fig. 8.9 Electrode array for facial nerve monitoring using the Nerve Integrity Monitor (NIM) (Medtronic Corp., Minneapolis, MN). There are two needle electrode pairs (*blue* and *red*) for live electromyographic (EMG) monitoring of the orbicularis oculi and orbicularis oris. A common ground electrode (*green*) completes the circuit. A second ground electrode (*white*) is used for monopolar stimulation. A sterile stimulator probe can be used to deliver current to the nerve during surgery.

surgery. The usual recording array uses one pair of needle electrodes in the orbicularis oculi muscle and a second pair in the orbicularis oris, plus a common ground (**Fig. 8.9**). A second ground electrode for the stimulator circuit is inserted into a distant location, usually the shoulder.

EMG monitoring produces various types of responses, and the surgeon needs to be familiar with these.[15,18] "Burst" responses are brief, nonrepetitive signals that occur in response to brief mechanical stimulation of the nerve (**Fig. 8.10A**). During surgery, burst responses will occur when one brushes against an exposed nerve with a blunt instrument. They serve as an immediate warning to the surgeon and do not usually forebode permanent injury unless the disturbing activity is forceful or sustained. "Train" responses are repetitive signals that occur in response to events that are longer in duration, such as mechanical traction on the nerve (**Fig. 8.10B**). The surgeon should cease whatever activity produced the train response to avoid permanent injury. Train responses also occur in response to thermal trauma, such as after saline irrigation. Direct electrical stimulation of the nerve elicits a "pulse" response, a synchronous repetitive signal (**Fig. 8.10C**). Each recording channel produces a different tone, so that the pulse responses are specific for the upper and lower divisions of the nerve.

Surgical Applications of Facial Nerve Stimulation/Monitoring

Primary Chronic Ear Surgery

In cholesteatoma surgery, facial nerve monitoring is most useful when dissecting disease away from an exposed facial nerve. As previously discussed, spontaneous bony dehiscences of the facial canal are common, and the incidence is higher in the presence of erosive disease. When a bare facial nerve is covered by cholesteatoma matrix or by granulation tissue, it is vulnerable to injury during the removal of the disease. The most common site of dehiscence is the tympanic segment of the nerve, just superior to the stapes (**Fig. 8.11**). The surgical strategy in these cases is to approach the nerve from posteriorly and superiorly, developing a plane of dissection between the intact bone and the mucosal layer, and lifting the matrix away from the surface of the bare nerve using a sharp instrument. Once this plane is established the disease will usually peel away, leaving the nerve sheath intact and undisturbed. In these cases, the nerve monitor will provide audible feedback if there is blunt or sharp disturbance (burst response) or if there is mechanical traction (train response). With careful surgical technique, no response will be elicited.

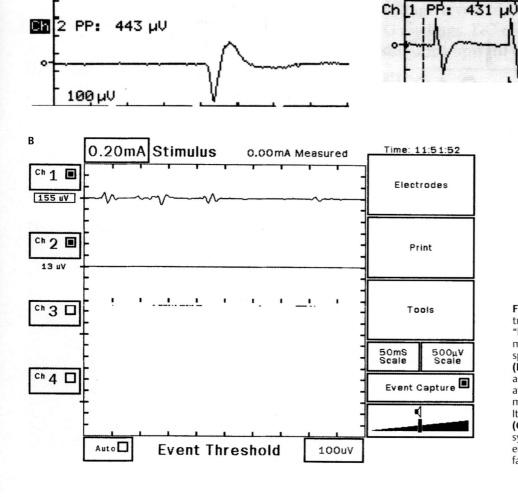

Fig. 8.10 Types of facial nerve electromyographic (EMG) responses. **(A)** A "burst" response is a brief, nonrepetitive muscle contraction and occurs in response to a direct mechanical stimulus. **(B)** A "train" response is a repetitive, asynchronous response that occurs after mechanical traction or prolonged mechanical stimulation of the nerve. It can also occur after cold irrigation. **(C)** A "pulse" response is a repetitive, synchronous compound action potential elicited by electrical stimulation of the facial nerve.

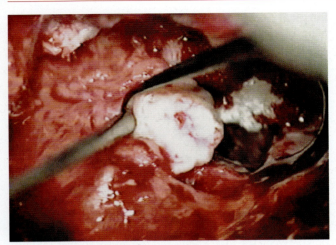

Fig. 8.11 Dissection of a recurrent cholesteatoma from bare facial nerve, tympanic segment, right ear, working from superiorly downward, using the stimulator probe as a dissecting instrument.

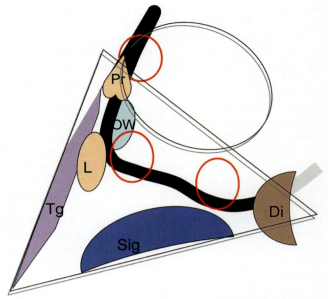

Fig. 8.12 Schematic view of the facial nerve (*black*), right ear. The three areas of vulnerability are indicated with red circles: at the facial recess, in the mastoid tip near the digastric (Di), and anterior to the process (Pr) in the anterior epitympanum. L, lateral semicircular canal; OW, oval window, Sig, sigmoid sinus; Tg, tegmen.

A second situation for monitoring may occur when one is drilling near the nerve, especially around the mastoid segment or second genu (**Fig. 8.12**). Although the nerve has a fairly constant anatomical course, variability exists in the medial-to-lateral position of the mastoid segment, approaching the digastric groove. Also, when opening the facial recess, it is desirable to shave away the bone anterior to the facial nerve to gain the best view of the sinus tympani (**Fig. 8.13**).

A third vulnerable area is anterior to the processus cochleariformis (**Fig. 8.12**), where the nerve may be exposed in the anterior epitympanic space. In these instances, the monitor may give a burst or train response if the drill or dissecting instrument brushes the nerve sheath. Injury may be avoided if the surgeon is aware of the slightly more lateral position of the nerve in this location.

In cases with distorted anatomy, or a nerve embedded in disease, the nerve stimulator may be used to map the course of the nerve anatomically. A monopolar stimulator, such as the Prass probe (Medtronic-Xomed Corp., Jacksonville, FL), can be used at a higher setting initially (eg, 2 mA) to verify that it is working, then the current setting can be turned down (0.5 mA) to gain more specific information about the position of the nerve. A bare nerve should stimulate briskly at 0.5 mA or less, whereas a nerve with an intact bony sheath will require more current, typically 2 mA or higher.

The stimulator can also be used after a difficult dissection to verify the integrity of the nerve. Stimulation with a suprathreshold current level proximal to the site of concern will produce a brisk response if the nerve is intact. An absent response or a very high threshold may be a reason to explore the nerve proximally and distally and to decompress the bony sheath.

Certain caveats should be noted during monitoring. Bipolar or monopolar electrocoagulation causes an artifactual response. This can be defeated using a muting circuit, but monitoring is suspended when muting is in effect. Irrigation can elicit a train response because of thermal stimulation of the nerve. Although this is not clinically significant, it may take several minutes for the response to die down and for normal monitoring to resume. Brief mechanical trauma using blunt dissecting instruments or

drill will cause a burst response—this is moderately significant and should be taken as a warning of impending injury if the activity that caused the response is not stopped. An instantaneous trauma to the nerve, however, may not elicit any response if it is very short in duration; therefore it is possible to have a serious injury to the nerve, such as sharp transection, without any signal at all from the nerve monitor.

Chronic Ear Disease Presenting with Facial Nerve Paralysis

When the patient has preoperative facial nerve paralysis in the presence of cholesteatoma or chronic inflammatory middle ear disease, the facial nerve stimulator/monitor is helpful for assessing the degree and location of injury. However, if the

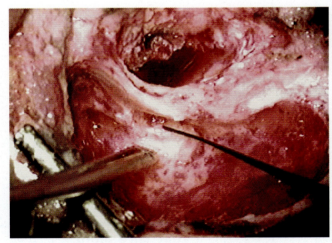

Fig. 8.13 Stimulation of the facial nerve in the facial recess (right ear).

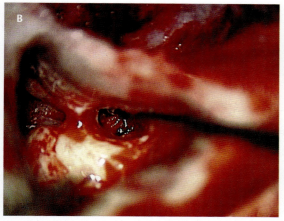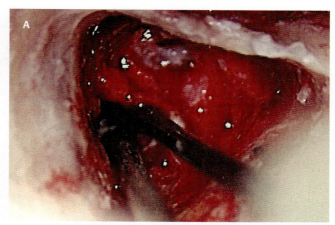

Fig. 8.14 Chronic suppurative otitis media of the right ear with acute facial paralysis. **(A)** Dissection of granulation tissue away from the tympanic segment of the facial nerve through the attic, using the stimulation probe. **(B)** After completion of the dissection, the nerve is stimulated along its length to test its function.

nerve does not respond to stimulation preoperatively, the device will not necessarily signal any further trauma to the nerve that occurs during the course of surgery.

After dissection of the disease, the exposed area of the nerve is visualized, and the bony covering is carefully removed proximal to the site of involvement (**Figs. 8.14A,B**). The presence of a response to electrical stimulation indicates that the nerve has functional integrity and will probably recover fully. The absence of a response, on the other hand, implies severe neuropraxia and a poorer prognosis, and the surgeon may want to decompress the nerve more widely to allow for progressive edema.

Postoperative Facial Nerve Paralysis

When the patient wakes up with immediate facial paralysis after chronic ear surgery, the patient is usually brought back to surgery for exploration and possible repair of the injured nerve. In this situation, the nerve monitor may be helpful for mapping the exact site of injury and indicating whether the disruption is complete or partial.

If the disruption is complete, the nerve edges should be freshened and the nerve reapproximated without tension using fine sutures (eg, 9–0 Prolene, Ethicon, Inc., Somerville, NJ). If the ends of the nerve cannot be brought together without tension, a nerve graft should be placed, using the great auricular nerve or sural nerve as a donor. If there is partial disruption, judgment must be used as to whether to allow the nerve to heal spontaneously or to repair the nerve primarily. If the injury involves less than a 50% cross-sectional area, or if the electrical response is preserved, the frayed edges of the nerve can be brought together with a collagen sheath, and partial recovery of function can be expected over a 6- to 12-month period.

Other Surgical Scenarios

If a middle ear tumor is suspected, the nerve monitor plays a valuable role because the anatomy may be altered and facial

nerve involvement may not be predicted preoperatively. *Middle ear adenoma* (**Fig. 8.15**) may mimic inflammatory ear disease and may erode the bony covering and compress or distort the nerve anywhere along its course. *Salivary choristoma* (**Fig. 8.16**) is composed of heterotopic salivary tissue that can occur anywhere along the facial nerve. Facial nerve paralysis has been reported after biopsy of this unusual lesion, and the facial nerve monitor may help to prevent injury.[19]

Glomus tympanicum tumors arise along the course of the Jacobson nerve within the middle ear cleft; glomus jugulare (**Fig. 8.17**) and glomus vagale tumors may grow into the middle ear space via the jugular foramen. Removing these tumors usually requires a facial recess approach; jugulare tumors often require facial nerve transposition or a facial bridge technique to the hypotympanum.

Facial nerve schwannomas can occur along the entire length of the facial nerve, and while these rarely occur solely

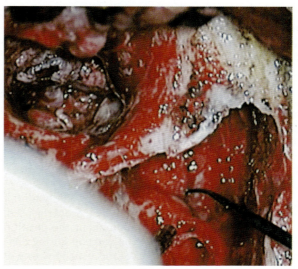

Fig. 8.15 Adenoma of the left middle ear and mastoid. The nerve stimulator probe is used to dissect the tumor away from the medial wall of the antrum approaching the facial nerve from posteriorly.

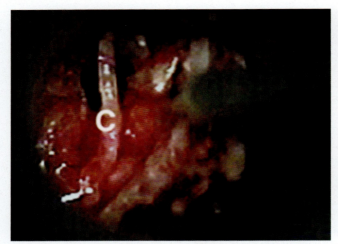

Fig. 8.16 Salivary choristoma of the middle ear, a rare entity consisting of heterotopic salivary tissue. The facial stimulator, seen here, can be used to be sure that the lesion does not stimulate before it is dissected. C, chorda tympani nerve.

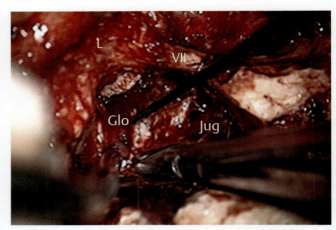

Fig. 8.17 Glomus jugulare tumor, right ear. A canal wall down mastoidectomy with facial bridge technique has been performed. The tumor (Glo) has been exposed in the retrofacial area, above the jugular bulb (Jug). L, lateral semicircular canal; VII, facial nerve.

in the middle ear, middle ear involvement is common. Removal of a facial nerve schwannoma will usually result in facial nerve paralysis, and primary grafting should be planned. If the diagnosis is not made preoperatively, the facial nerve stimulator can be helpful for confirming the fact that the tumor is of facial nerve origin.

Issues and Controversies Regarding Facial Nerve Monitoring

Debate continues over whether or not to routinely monitor the facial nerve during chronic ear surgery. Unlike acoustic neuroma surgery, where most surgeons would consider facial nerve monitoring to be indispensable, in chronic ear surgery the issue is less clearly resolved.

The incidence of facial nerve paralysis in routine mastoidectomy is low, even in the presence of cholesteatoma. Some surgeons would argue that the surgical anatomy is familiar, and using a monitor does not reduce the chance of facial nerve injury. Indeed, monitoring will not necessarily warn against sudden, penetrating injury, as already discussed. And in inexperienced hands, the nerve monitor may contribute to a false sense of security leading to a surgical misadventure. Proper training in the setup and use of facial nerve monitoring is therefore essential. Further, monitoring has a significant monetary cost—a commercially made unit costs around $20,000.00, the disposable electrodes up to $100.00 for each use, and a disposable stimulator probe even more. Some centers use a technician for live monitoring, adding to the cost. The increased time for setup creates intangible costs as well.

On the other hand, it is easy to argue for the potential benefits of facial nerve monitoring. When properly used, the monitor gives valuable information about the position of the nerve, provides feedback to the surgeon during delicate dissection on an exposed nerve, and usually warns of impending injury. These benefits would be difficult to prove "scientifically" because the variables encountered in surgery do not lend themselves easily to quantitative measurement

in an outcome study, but most surgeons would agree that the information provided by monitoring could help prevent a facial nerve complication. Because the incidence of facial nerve injury is very low, a very large study would have to be constructed to have sufficient statistical power. Facial paralysis will often result in medicolegal action, even in the absence of negligence or wrongdoing by the surgeon,[20] and failing to use a nerve monitor may be perceived as a departure from current "best practices."

In real-world current practice, the facial nerve monitor is probably used by most surgeons in most cases of cholesteatoma surgery. Although some surgeons will employ it selectively, monitoring should probably be set up and used routinely to be most useful because it is impossible to predict when it will really be needed.[21] In a policy statement,[22] the American Academy of Otolaryngology–Head and Neck Surgery (AAO-HNS) has recognized "the proven efficacy of neurophysiologic monitoring of the facial nerve which may minimize the risk of injury to the nerve during surgical procedures in which the nerve is vulnerable." But they also state that these "guidelines are not a substitute for the experience and judgment of a physician . . . and in no sense do they represent a standard of care." This statement strikes a balance between the opinions of surgeons' pro and con.

◆ Endoscopes in Chronic Ear Surgery

Endoscopes have proved to be a useful adjunct to surgery of the middle ear and mastoid.[23] The advantage provided by the endoscope is the ability to place the surgeon's eye deep within the surgical cavity, and to be able to look around corners. This provides an advantage in areas such as the facial recess and anterior epitympanic space, which are difficult to visualize directly using the microscope. The disadvantages of the endoscope are the need to switch from the microscope to a different optical system (using a separate video setup or the naked eye), the presence of an object within the surgical field (with the potential to injure the stapes or facial nerve), the generation of heat (another potential source of injury),

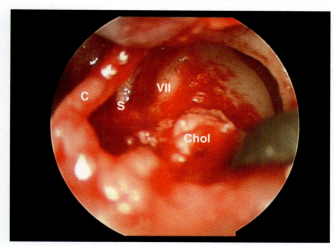

Fig. 8.18 Endoscopic view of left ear showing residual cholesteatoma in the attic and posterior tympanic sinus that was not seen with the microscope alone. C, chorda tympani; VII, facial nerve; S, stapes; Chol, cholesteatoma.

the loss of three-dimensionality, the loss of a free hand (or the need for an assistant to hold the scope), and the loss of visualization while operating with blood in the surgical field. These disadvantages make it unlikely that the endoscope will replace the microscope in ear surgery, but the enhanced visualization makes the endoscope useful nonetheless.

Smaller endoscopes provide a view of recesses within the middle ear space. A 2.7 mm, 30 degree scope can be inserted into the middle ear via a tympanomeatal flap, allowing the surgeon to look in the sinus tympani and epitympanum and reducing the possibility of leaving disease behind. This should translate into a lower rate of residual disease, and some authors have claimed improved results.[24,25] The ability to peer around corners may also permit less bone removal during mastoid surgery. It is possible that the endoscope may preclude the need for a facial recess approach for sinus tympani disease, allowing the surgeon to look in the sinus tympani and epitympanum and reducing the possibility of leaving disease behind (**Fig. 8.18**).[26]

The endoscope may also allow for a less invasive approach for second-stage surgery.[27,28] Passing the endoscope through a small stab incision in the postauricular scar allows the surgeon to rule out residual disease in the mastoid cavity without the need for a large postauricular incision (but of course if disease is found, a formal revision operation will be necessary).

An endoscope-only technique has been devised for surgery of the middle ear and attic.[29] Using a 4 mm endoscope in the ear canal gives a wider field of view than the microscope can, and allows a complete transcanal atticotomy to be performed. For disease confined to the attic, this may provide thorough surgical removal through a more limited approach.

◆ Adequacy of Follow-Up

Adequacy of follow-up is an important factor in determining success or failure after cholesteatoma surgery. Follow-up is necessary to determine whether a patient has recurrent or

residual disease, to clean and to manage problem cavities, and to assess postoperative hearing status in the short and long term. In clinical practice, however, many factors affect the reliability of follow-up, such as the patient's distance from the surgeon, (changeable) insurance status, relationship with a referring physician, or moving out of the area. Without regular follow-up, the long-term results of cholesteatoma management are unknowable. For surgeons with out-of-town referral sources, this can be an even greater problem.

The tendency of cholesteatoma to recur lends particular importance to this issue. In a patient whose reliability is in question, CWD surgery is often the safest option. CWD has an intrinsically low recurrence rate, and residual disease can be spotted on exam and often dealt with in an office setting. Further, CWD exteriorizes the mastoid, so that complications (ie, spread of infection to the labyrinth, facial nerve, or intracranial structures) are unlikely to occur.

Several studies have taken up the issue as to what constitutes adequate length of follow-up. The recurrence rate for cholesteatoma increases with the length of follow-up in both children and adults.[30-32] Because cholesteatoma is thought to be more aggressive disease in children, the importance of follow-up is greater in pediatric patients. Recurrent cholesteatoma can form at any time, even years after the original surgical procedure (in contrast to residual disease, which is theoretically present at the conclusion of the surgery). Long-term follow-up studies have reported recurrent disease up to 15 years later, and giant cholesteatomas have been discovered after even longer intervals.[33] Although the likelihood of recurrence diminishes with time, there is no end point, practically speaking, at which follow-up is no longer needed.

The reporting of results can be influenced by the adequacy of follow-up. This can affect the surgeon's perceived success rate in treating patients. Most studies traditionally used a standard rate calculation, where the total number of observed recurrences is divided by the total number of years of follow-up for the study. This method, however, fails to account for patients who drop from follow-up, or who have insufficient length of follow-up.[34] The use of Kaplan-Meier analysis adjusts for those who are "censored" from the study, and gives a truer estimate of disease recurrence overall.[35]

◆ Conclusions

1. Canal wall up and canal wall down operations each play an important role in the management of cholesteatoma, and factors including mastoid size, aggressiveness of disease, presence of complications, and reliability of follow-up should be considered in selecting the best approach in a given patient. Reconstructed canal wall techniques may provide a useful compromise in certain cases.
2. Second-stage surgery can be useful in certain patients to rule out recurrent or residual disease and to allow for ossicular chain reconstruction in a stable middle ear.
3. Facial nerve stimulation and monitoring provide an added measure of patient safety but do not replace surgical judgment, anatomical knowledge, or technical skill.

4. Endoscopes may play a useful role in the management of sinus tympani disease and in the detection of recurrence using a minimally invasive approach.
5. Adequacy of follow-up is an important factor in cholesteatoma management because the recurrence rate remains significant, even in the most experienced hands.

References

1. Mosher HP. A method of filling the excavated mastoid with a flap from the back of the auricle. Laryngoscope 1911;21:1158–1163
2. Wullstein SR. Osteoplastic epitympanotomy: tympanoplasty types I, II, III: a review of 15 years of experience. Am J Otol 1985;6(1):5–8
3. Silvola J, Palva T. Pediatric one-stage cholesteatoma surgery: long term results. Int J Pediatr Otorhinolaryngol 1999;49(suppl 1):S87–S90
4. Roberson JB Jr, Mason TP, Stidham KR. Mastoid obliteration: autogenous cranial bone pAte reconstruction. Otol Neurotol 2003;24(2):132–140
5. Mercke U. The cholesteatomatous ear one year after surgery with obliteration technique. Am J Otol 1987;8(6):534–536
6. Gantz BJ, Wilkinson EP, Hansen MR. Canal wall reconstruction tympanomastoidectomy with mastoid obliteration. Laryngoscope 2005;115(10):1734–1740
7. McElveen JT Jr, Chung ATA. Reversible canal wall down mastoidectomy for acquired cholesteatomas: preliminary results. Laryngoscope 2003;113(6):1027–1033
8. Smith PG, Stroud MH, Goebel JA. Soft-wall reconstruction of the posterior external ear canal wall. Otolaryngol Head Neck Surg 1986;94(3):355–359
9. Takahashi H, Iwanaga T, Kaieda S, et al. Mastoid obliteration combined with soft-wall reconstruction of posterior ear canal. Eur Arch Otorhinolaryngol 2007;264(8):867–871
10. Dornhoffer JL. Retrograde mastoidectomy with canal wall reconstruction: a follow-up report. Otol Neurotol 2004;25(5):653–660
11. Mahendran S, Yung MW. Mastoid obliteration with hydroxyapatite cement: the Ipswich experience. Otol Neurotol 2004;25(1):19–21
12. Grote JJ. Results of cavity reconstruction with hydroxyapatite implants after 15 years. Am J Otol 1998;19(5):565–568
13. Della Santina CC, Lee SC. Ceravital reconstruction of canal wall down mastoidectomy: long-term results. Arch Otolaryngol Head Neck Surg 2006;132(6):617–623
14. Sudhoff H, Brors D, Al-Lawati A, Gimenez E, Dazert S, Hildmann H. Posterior canal wall reconstruction with a composite cartilage titanium mesh graft in canal wall down tympanoplasty and revision surgery for radical cavities. J Laryngol Otol 2006;120(10):832–836
15. Niparko JK, Kileny PR, Kemink JL, Lee HM, Graham MD. Neurophysiologic intraoperative monitoring, II: Facial nerve function. Am J Otol 1989;10(1):55–61
16. Smouha EE. Facial nerve monitoring and stimulation during surgery for chronic ear disease. Operative Techniques in Otolaryngol 1992;3:43–47
17. Kartush JM, Niparko JK, Bledsoe SC, Graham MD, Kemink JL. Intraoperative facial nerve monitoring: a comparison of stimulating electrodes. Laryngoscope 1985;95(12):1536–1540
18. Prass RL, Lüders H. Acoustic (loudspeaker) facial electromyographic monitoring, I: Evoked electromyographic activity during acoustic neuroma resection. Neurosurgery 1986;19(3):392–400
19. Namdar I, Smouha EE, Kane P. Salivary gland choristoma of the middle ear: role of intraoperative facial nerve monitoring. Otolaryngol Head Neck Surg 1995;112(4):616–620
20. Lydiatt DD. Medical malpractice and facial nerve paralysis. Arch Otolaryngol Head Neck Surg 2003;129(1):50–53
21. Silverstein H, Smouha E, Jones R. Routine identification of the facial nerve using electrical stimulation during otological and neurotological surgery. Laryngoscope 1988;98(7):726–730
22. American Academy of Otolaryngology–Head and Neck Surgery. Policy Statement on Facial Nerve Monitoring. Available at: www.entnet.org/Practice/policyFacialNerveMonitoring.cfm
23. Rosenberg SI, Silverstein H, Willcox TO, Gordon MA. Endoscopy in otology and neurotology. Am J Otol 1994;15(2):168–172
24. Thomassin JM, Korchia D, Doris JM. Endoscopic-guided otosurgery in the prevention of residual cholesteatomas. Laryngoscope 1993;103(8):939–943
25. Yung MW. The use of middle ear endoscopy: has residual cholesteatoma been eliminated? J Laryngol Otol 2001;115(12):958–961
26. Marchioni D, Mattioli F, Alicandri-Ciufelli M, Presutti L. Transcanal endoscopic approach to the sinus tympani: a clinical report. Otol Neurotol 2009;30(6):758–765
27. McKennan KX. Endoscopic 'second look' mastoidoscopy to rule out residual epitympanic/mastoid cholesteatoma. Laryngoscope 1993;103(7):810–814
28. Haberkamp TJ, Tanyeri H. Surgical techniques to facilitate endoscopic second-look mastoidectomy. Laryngoscope 1999;109(7 Pt 1):1023–1027
29. Tarabichi M. Endoscopic management of limited attic cholesteatoma. Laryngoscope 2004;114(7):1157–1162
30. Parisier SC, Hanson MB, Han JC, Cohen AJ, Selkin BA. Pediatric cholesteatoma: an individualized, single-stage approach. Otolaryngol Head Neck Surg 1996;115(1):107–114
31. Lau T, Tos M. Cholesteatoma in children: recurrence related to observation period. Am J Otolaryngol 1987;8(6):364–375
32. Tos M, Lau T. Attic cholesteatoma: recurrence rate related to observation time. Am J Otol 1988;9(6):456–464
33. Geven LI, Mulder JJ, Graamans K. Giant cholesteatoma: recommendations for follow-up. Skull Base 2008;18(5):353–359
34. Mishiro Y, Sakagami M, Kitahara T, Kondoh K, Okumura S. The investigation of the recurrence rate of cholesteatoma using Kaplan-Meier survival analysis. Otol Neurotol 2008;29(6):803–806
35. Stangerup SE, Drozdziewicz D, Tos M, Hougaard-Jensen A. Recurrence of attic cholesteatoma: different methods of estimating recurrence rates. Otolaryngol Head Neck Surg 2000;123(3):283–287

9

Congenital Cholesteatoma

Congenital cholesteatoma is cholesteatoma that occurs in a child, behind an intact tympanic membrane.[1] Congenital cholesteatoma is thought to arise from an epithelial rest that gets trapped in the middle ear cleft in utero, and that enlarges over time to form a ball of keratinizing squamous epithelium.[2] This entity is truly, then, an epidermoid tumor, rather than the end-product of an inflammatory process, although Tos has argued the contrary.[3]

Congenital cholesteatomas are usually discovered in infants or young children on routine physical exam. They appear as a white mass behind an intact tympanic membrane (**Fig. 9.1**). The average age at presentation is ~4 years. In the original description of congenital cholesteatoma by Derlacki and Clemis,[4] the diagnosis required that the ear be otherwise completely normal, with no history of otitis media. Because the incidence of otitis media is high in the general population of children, however, a history of ear infection or the presence of a middle ear effusion should not disqualify the diagnosis, as long as there is no history of otorrhea and the tympanic membrane is free of perforation or retraction. In fact, a certain number of congenital cholesteatomas will first be discovered during a myringotomy for serous otitis.

Congenital cholesteatomas begin in the middle ear in two general locations—in the anterosuperior quadrant (**Fig. 9.1**) or in the posterosuperior quadrant. The former are usually associated with an intact ossicular chain and, if detected early enough, can be removed completely with the expectation of a normal hearing outcome. The latter often involve the incus and stapes early and are less likely to result in normal hearing. Congenital cholesteatomas that are missed in early childhood and that are allowed to become sizable will behave no differently from acquired cholesteatomas—they will erode bone as they grow, and they will eventually perforate and drain.[5] Congenital cholesteatomas are almost always unilateral; however, bilateral congenital cholesteatomas have been described.[6]

The treatment of congenital cholesteatoma is surgical. These should be operated on when first discovered, to prevent the potential problems associated with continued growth.

Anteriorly situated cholesteatomas can usually be removed via an extended tympanotomy approach, as described by Levenson et al.[1] A transmeatal approach can usually be employed, even in younger children, but it is acceptable to use a postauricular incision to gain adequate exposure if the meatus is very small. A standard tympanomeatal incision is made in the posterior canal skin, and is extended anteriorly to ~3 o'clock in the right ear, or 9 o'clock in the left ear, to create a flap that is pedicled to the anterior-inferior canal skin (**Fig. 9.2**). After elevating the flap, the drum is separated from the manubrium of the malleus (**Fig. 9.3**). This is the key step in gaining anterior exposure. This is done by incising the investing mucosa along the length of the malleus with a sharp pick and peeling the drum epithelium downward, like a stocking, toward the umbo. The fibrous insertion of the drum to the umbo can be incised with a Bellucci scissors—this allows the flap to be reflected forward and downward to gain maximal exposure of the anterior middle ear space.

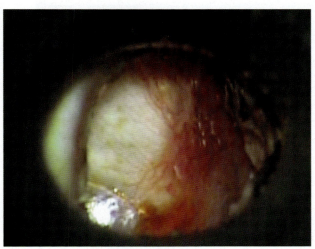

Fig. 9.1 Congenital cholesteatoma: otoscopic view of a white mass in the anterosuperior quadrant of the left ear.

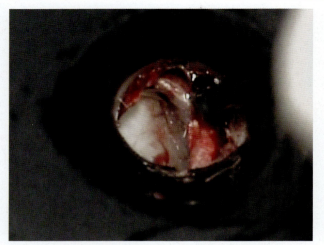

Fig. 9.2 Tympanomeatal incision is extended anteriorly to 9 o'clock (for left ear), creating a flap that will be pedicled anteroinferiorly.

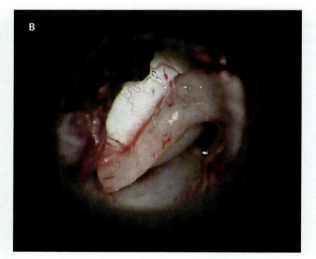

Fig. 9.3 The mucosa is incised along the length of the malleus, and the drum is separated from the malleus working from above downward. The umbo is detached using Bellucci scissors.

This approach should be sufficient to expose the anterior and inferior margins of the cholesteatoma sac (**Fig. 9.4A,B**).

The superior margin may extend upward to the attic and can be exposed by removing the edge of the scutum with

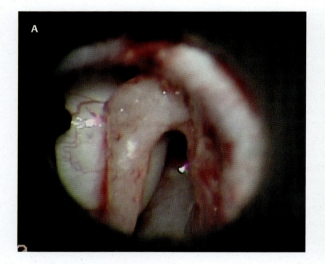

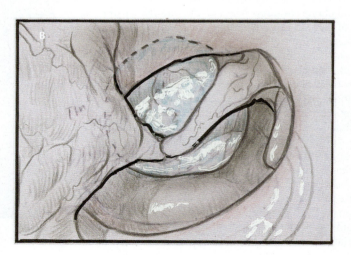

Fig. 9.4 With the extended tympanomeatal flap lifted forward, the entire cholesteatoma can be seen. **(A)** The anterior and superior, and **(B)** the interior and posterior extent of the lesion are visualized.

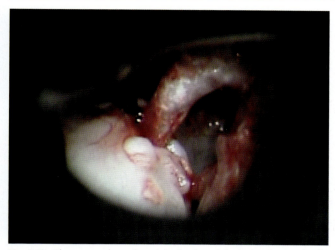

Fig. 9.5 The mucosal envelope is incised, and the lesion is completely mobilized.

a stapes curette. The cholesteatoma is enveloped by a very thin layer of normal mucosa. This mucosal layer is incised along the inferior margin of the sac, and the lesion is freed by blunt dissection using a sweeping motion with a whirlybird (Hough excavator) along the anterior and superior borders, keeping the capsule intact (**Fig. 9.5**). The lesion is usually attached to the tensor tympani tendon near the processus, and should be separated sharply from the tensor using a Rosen needle. The cholesteatoma can usually be delivered in toto once this is done.

Occasionally the lesion cannot be removed without rupturing the sac. If this does occur, the contents (debris) should be carefully evacuated with suction and cup forceps, care being taken not to spill the contents of the lesion into the middle ear, and the capsule should be maintained as completely as possible on the medial (deep) surface. Once the lesion is reduced in size, the capsule can be dissected and the remainder of the sac delivered.

Once the lesion is removed, it is important to inspect the attic and protympanum using a mirror or endoscope to be sure that there is no residual disease (**Fig. 9.6A–C**). It is also

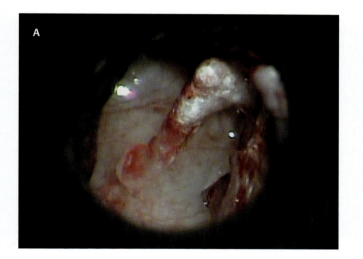

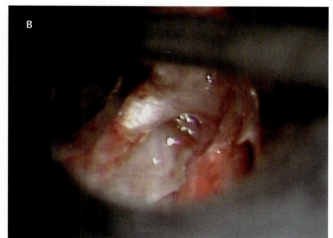

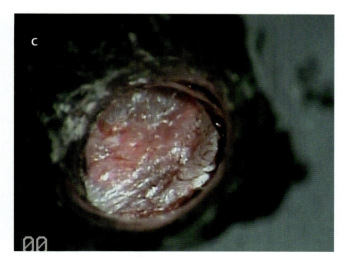

Fig. 9.6 **(A,B)** The lesion is completely removed. A mirror is used to inspect the tensor tendon, processus, and anterior surface of the malleus to ensure that no epithelium remains. **(C)** The tympanomeatal flap is returned.

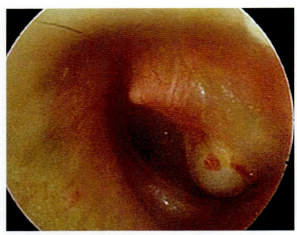

Fig. 9.7 Endoscopic photograph of posteriorly situated congenital cholesteatoma of the left ear.

advisable to scrape the anterior surface of the tensor tendon with a sharp pick to be certain that no epithelium is left there. The tympanomeatal flap can be replaced and the external canal packed lightly with Gelfoam (Pfizer, Inc., New York, NY). The ear should heal normally, with normal hearing resulting.

Posteriorly situated cholesteatomas (**Fig. 9.7**) cannot usually be removed in toto because they usually involve the incus. In this respect they must be handled more like acquired cholesteatomas. After an extended tympanomeatal flap is raised (**Fig. 9.8A,B**), the posterior and superior bony overhang is removed with a curette, and the extent of the lesion is evaluated (**Fig. 9.9A,B**). The incus must usually be separated from the stapes and removed if it is enveloped by the disease (**Fig. 9.10A,B**). If there is considerable superior extension to the epitympanum (**Fig. 9.11**), a transcanal atticotomy can be performed, removing the scutum with a curette until the posterosuperior margin is identified. The sac is dissected from the medial attic wall toward the middle ear and delivered (**Figs. 9.11** and **9.12**). Primary ossicular recon-

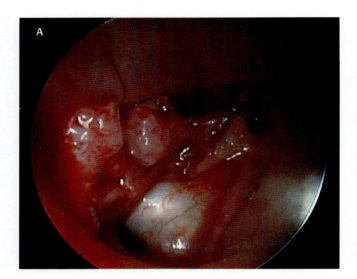

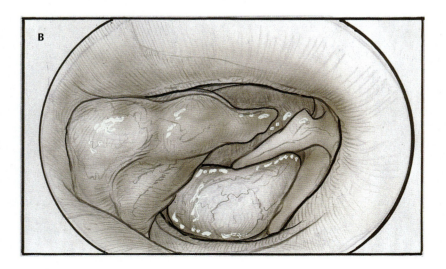

Fig. 9.8 **(A,B)** Extended tympanomeatal flap. The incision is carried toward 9 o'clock (3 o'clock for a right ear), and the drum is separated from the malleus, allowing anterior exposure.

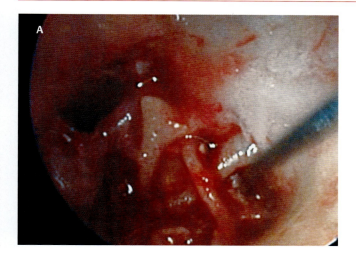

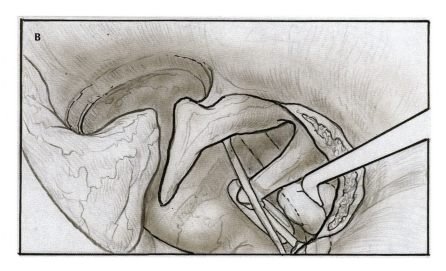

Fig. 9.9 **(A,B)** After curetting the posterosuperior bony overhang, the posterior aspect of the sac can be dissected forward. The sac travels medial to the incus.

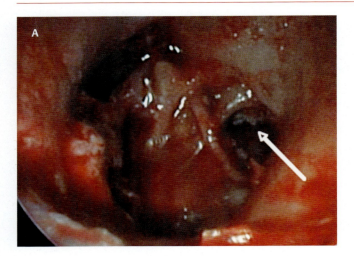

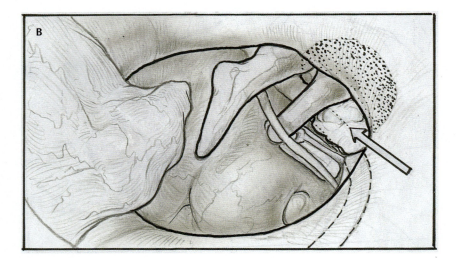

Fig. 9.10 **(A,B)** The disease extends to the epitympanum (*arrow*). The incus will have to be removed, as well as part of the scutum, to gain adequate exposure.

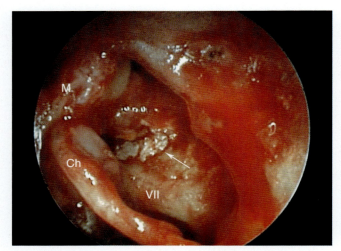

Fig. 9.11 The incus is removed and the atticotomy performed. There is residual disease on the medial attic wall (*arrow*). M, malleus head; VII, facial nerve; Ch, chorda tympani.

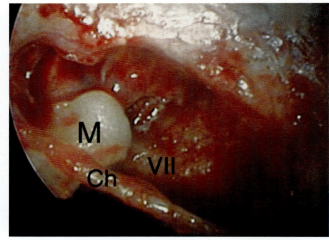

Fig. 9.12 Endoscopic view of the attic, showing all disease removed. M, malleus head; VII, facial nerve; Ch, chorda tympani.

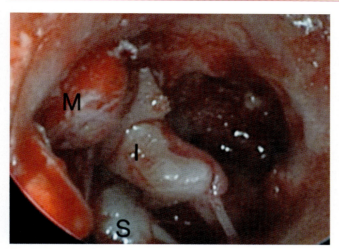

Fig. 9.13 Ossicular reconstruction using a sculpted incus (I) interposed between the malleus (M) and stapes (S).

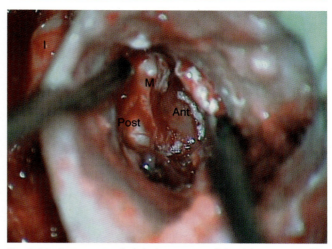

Fig. 9.14 Large congenital cholesteatoma of the right ear treated by canal wall up mastoidectomy. Disease was dissected out of the antrum from around the incus (I) and delivered toward the middle ear. A posterior mesotympanic component (Post) and a shell of anterior mesotympanic component (Ant) remain. M, malleus.

struction can be undertaken, as shown here, or delayed until a second stage (**Fig. 9.13**).

Large congenital cholesteatomas are handled in the same way as large acquired cholesteatomas. A canal wall up mastoidectomy is created to assess the posterior extent of the disease. A transcanal atticotomy is performed to remove the disease from the epitympanum, and a facial recess opening to dissect the sac from the posterior mesotympanum (**Fig. 9.14**). If the exposure is still restricted, a decision can be made intraoperatively to convert this to a canal wall down mastoidectomy.

References

1. Levenson MJ, Michaels L, Parisier SC. Congenital cholesteatomas of the middle ear in children: origin and management. Otolaryngol Clin North Am 1989;22(5):941–954

2. Michaels L. Origin of congenital cholesteatoma from a normally occurring epidermoid rest in the developing middle ear. Int J Pediatr Otorhinolaryngol 1988;15(1):51–65

3. Tos M. A new pathogenesis of mesotympanic (congenital) cholesteatoma. Laryngoscope 2000;110(11):1890–1897

4. Derlacki EL, Clemis JD. Congenital cholesteatoma of the middle ear and mastoid. Ann Otol Rhinol Laryngol 1965;74(3):706–727

5. Grundfast KM, Ahuja GS, Parisier SC, Culver SM. Delayed diagnosis and fate of congenital cholesteatoma (keratoma). Arch Otolaryngol Head Neck Surg 1995;121(8):903–907

6. Litman RS, Smouha E, Sher WH, Shangold LM. Two cases of bilateral congenital cholesteatoma—usual and unusual presentations. Int J Pediatr Otorhinolaryngol 1996;36(3):241–252

10

Recidivism

The possibility of disease recurrence makes the surgical management of cholesteatoma challenging. *Recurrent* cholesteatoma is defined as cholesteatoma that re-forms after complete surgical excision. *Residual* cholesteatoma is disease left behind by the surgeon. *Recidivism* refers to the combination of recurrent and residual disease. The rate of recurrent disease after canal wall up surgery is high, ~20%, and may be even higher in children.[1,2]

◆ Recurrent Cholesteatoma

Recurrent disease may form after canal wall up mastoidectomy and occasionally after canal wall down procedures. In contrast to residual cholesteatoma, recurrent disease occurs when a retraction pocket re-forms from the tympanic membrane, extending upward to the attic or backward toward the sinus tympani. Failure to reconstruct the scutum after intact canal wall mastoidectomy can provide a space for recurrence to form, but disease may recur even when the scutum is rebuilt with cartilage at the initial operation.[3] This may begin by invagination of tympanic membrane epithelium into the middle ear space, which can then extend back to the attic and later the mastoid. In other cases, the recurrence may erode the scutum or the posterior bony canal wall and extend superiorly.

Recognition of recurrent disease is not always easy. In cases in which the scutum was originally reconstructed with cartilage, the recurrent cholesteatoma may begin in the space between the cartilage graft and the bony scutum, and the opening of the sac may not be apparent. Examination under the microscope is the single best method of detecting recurrent cholesteatoma. A retraction pocket can be gently probed with a blunt hook to determine its depth and whether it contains squamous material. The case shown in **Fig. 10.1A** is a patient with a canal wall up operation for attic cholesteatoma with cartilage graft reconstruction of the scutum, who complained only of fullness, without hearing loss or discharge. Gentle probing revealed the scutum defect to be part of a deep sac. The operative findings are shown

in the **Fig. 10.1B**, a recurrent cholesteatoma extending from attic to antrum. This was managed by canal wall down mastoidectomy with bony obliteration of the mastoid cavity (**Fig. 10.1C,D**). She has remained free of recurrence for 4 years.

Recurrent cholesteatoma can also form in the middle ear. Retraction pockets that redevelop in the pars tensa typically grow either upward, toward the attic, or medially and backward, toward the sinus tympani (**Fig. 10.2**).

The endoscope can be a useful tool for detecting a recurrence in the office. By allowing illumination deep in the cavity, and by putting the viewer's eye close to the area of interest, the endoscope may allow the physician to look into crevices and around bony obstructions and see more than can be appreciated with the microscope. The case shown in **Fig. 10.3** is an endoscopic view of the right ear of a young girl who had undergone a canal wall up mastoidectomy with staged middle ear reconstruction by another surgeon. She complained of hearing decline after initial hearing gain. On otomicroscopic exam, the meatus was constricted and there was middle ear collapse, but the attic could not be adequately assessed. With endoscopy, squamous material could be seen in the attic, under the ledge of bone, signifying regrowth of cholesteatoma (**Fig. 10.3A**). At surgery, there was a very large recurrent cholesteatoma filling the attic, and a canal wall down procedure was performed (**Fig. 10.3B**).

The presence of recurring discharge and polyp, especially in the absence of a tympanic membrane perforation, should suggest the presence of recurrence even when a retraction pocket and/or squamous debris are not evident. Declining hearing in ears with good initial postoperative hearing is also suggestive of recurrence. The case illustrated in **Fig. 10.4** is a 6-year-old child who underwent canal wall up mastoidectomy with total ossicular replacement prosthesis (TORP) reconstruction of the middle ear, with an excellent hearing result. After 9 months the hearing declined. Microscopic evaluation revealed pars tensa collapse (**Fig. 10.4A**) but endoscopic exam showed a large retraction pocket extending to the attic (**Fig. 10.4B**). A canal wall down mastoidectomy was performed.

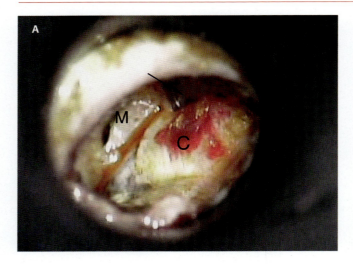

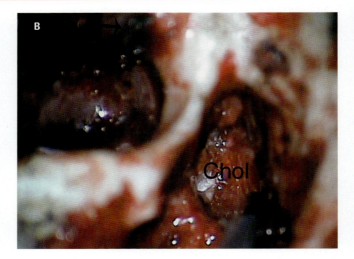

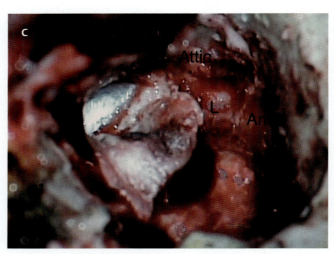

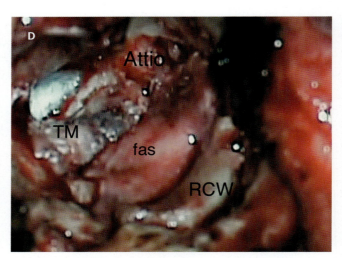

Fig. 10.1 **(A)** The patient had undergone left canal wall up mastoidectomy with cartilage graft **(C)** reconstruction of the scutum and had declining hearing and ear fullness. The patient had a stable attic retraction pocket (*arrow*) without drainage or squamous debris. (M = malleus) **(B)** At surgery, a moderately large cholesteatoma (Chol) is filling the posterior epitympanum and extending to the antrum. **(C)** Canal wall down mastoidectomy, with disease completely excised. The canal wall was removed en bloc. L, lateral semicircular canal; Antr, antrum. **(D)** The middle ear was reconstructed with a type 3 tympanoplasty (tympanic membrane on stapes head). The posterior canal bone was replaced to create a reconstructed canal wall (RCW). The attic was left open to prevent further recurrence, and fascia (fas) was used to reline the base of the cavity.

Computed tomographic (CT) scan can be helpful, particularly when the original procedure was done by another surgeon. In the case of prior intact wall mastoidectomy, the scan demonstrates the size of the mastoid and the extent of bone removal. It also might show the presence of neocortical bone formation, and anatomical areas that might have been left unexplored during the original procedure. CT also demonstrates the presence or absence of ossicles. CT is useful in predicting a complication, such as a lateral semicircular canal fistula or dehiscent tegmen, and may prevent problems during revision surgery. In the case of prior canal wall down mastoidectomy, CT shows the remaining bony anatomy, and possible shortcomings of prior surgery, such as a high facial ridge and retained mastoid. For example, **Fig. 10.5** shows a CT image of a patient with a recurrent cholesteatoma that had grown through a tight attic defect in a canal wall down mastoid cavity. CT, however, might not always prove the diagnosis of recurrent cholesteatoma.

Cholesteatoma appears as a soft tissue density on CT scan but may be indistinguishable from inflamed mucosa, granulation tissue, or retained fluid. Residual disease may appear

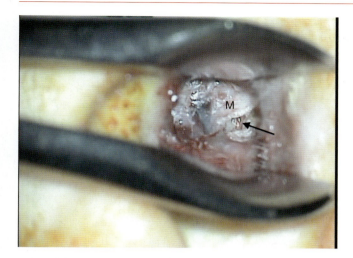

Fig. 10.2 A middle ear recurrence of the left ear, in the posterosuperior quadrant (*arrow*). M, malleus.

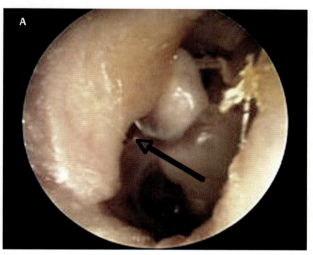

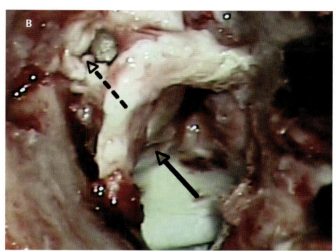

Fig. 10.3 Recurrent cholesteatoma of the right ear detected by endoscopy. **(A)** Endoscopic photo showing tympanic membrane collapsed onto the promontory and around TORP. There was squamous debris visible under the scutum ledge, in the direction of the *arrow*. **(B)** Surgical photo, showing large recurrent cholesteatoma in the mastoid cavity. The *arrows* show the same line of sight as in the endoscopic photo.

as a spherical density in a well pneumatized mastoid cavity (**Fig. 10.6**). In intact canal wall mastoidectomy, fibrous tissue often fills the mastoid cavity and also appears as a soft tissue density. This perfectly benign finding may be differentiated from recurrent cholesteatoma or other forms of inflammatory soft tissue by its concave margins, although this is not routinely true (**Fig. 10.7**). The use of magnetic resonance imaging (MRI) in conjunction with CT has been advocated by some as the means of establishing or disproving recurrence.[4] Diffusion-weighted MRI in particular appears to have a high positive and negative predictive value.[5] However, MRI is not routinely utilized in the clinical setting because scanning is expensive and subject to motion artifact, and surgery will

probably be recommended in highly suspicious cases regardless of the radiologic findings.

Revision Surgery for Recurrent Cholesteatoma in Canal Wall Up Cavity

The patient is prepped and draped in the same manner as for primary surgery. Lidocaine (1%) with epinephrine 1:100,000 is injected into the canal and postauricular skin for hemostasis. First the drum is examined through the meatus, debriding any pus and polyp from the ear canal. Usually the diagnosis

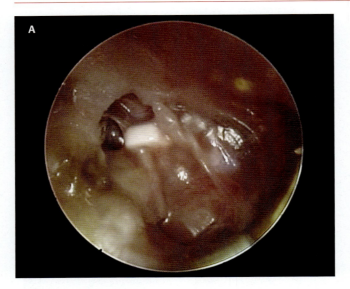
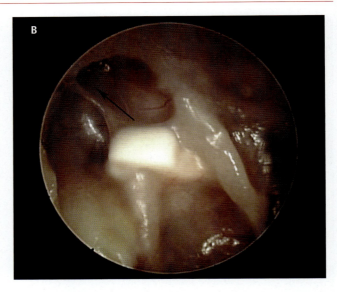

Fig. 10.4   Declining hearing after canal wall up mastoidectomy with TORP, right ear. **(A)** View from the external canal shows the pars tensa retracted around the prosthesis. **(B)** A deeper endoscopic view shows a large attic retraction, which required canal wall down revision mastoidectomy.

will be evident at this point if it could not be confirmed during office microscopy. Gentle probing may reveal bony defect in the scutum or posterior bony canal (**Fig. 10.8A**), and pressure on the soft tissue may express squamous debris, thereby confirming the diagnosis. Canal incisions should be made just lateral to the bony defect so as to maintain as much viable canal skin as possible for later reconstruction.

A postauricular incision is created, and the mastoid periosteum is incised posterior and superior to the bony mastoidectomy defect if possible. The fibrous tissue in the mastoid can then either be excavated directly from the depth of the cavity or incised at the plane of the mastoid cortex and left in place until after the canal skin is separated from the bone (the latter method allows for more control when dissecting

the tissue out of the mastoid). The superior periosteal incision should proceed along the temporal line and far enough anterior so that the anterior epitympanum can be accessed.

Bony exposure is obtained starting from the mastoid and working forward. In most revision mastoidectomy cases, if the disease fills the mastoid extensively, the posterior bony canal wall will almost certainly have to be removed. In cases in which the recurrent disease is localized to the attic, however, it may be possible to maintain the posterior canal wall. As in primary cases, it pays to begin the bony dissection posteriorly, preserving the canal wall at least initially. First the neocortical bony edges are removed and the tegmen mastoideum is identified. Posteriorly, the sigmoid sinus is identified and the retrosigmoid bone is removed. The tegmen is

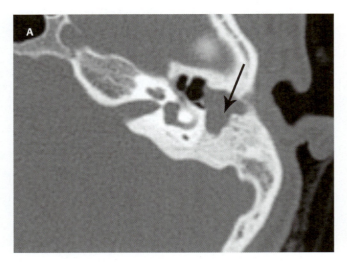
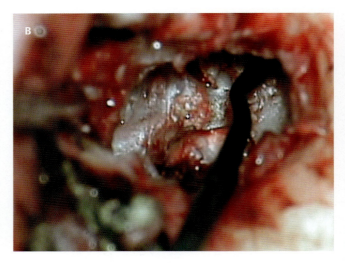

Fig. 10.5   Recurrent cholesteatoma in a contracted mastoid. **(A)** Computed tomographic scan demonstrates the recurrence pushed through a small atticotomy defect (*arrow*) to fill the mastoid antrum. **(B)** Surgical photo showing a recurrent cholesteatoma in the attic and antrum.

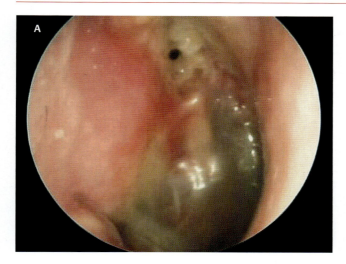 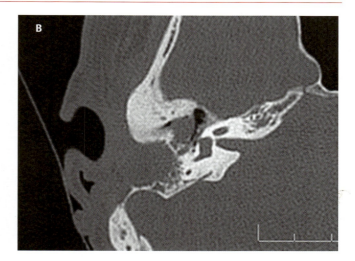

Fig. 10.6 Recurrent cholesteatoma, characterized by recurrent ear discharge. **(A)** On otoscopic exam, the drum appeared normal, whereas endoscopy revealed a tiny attic perforation that expelled pus on Valsalva. **(B)** Computed tomography showed a spherical tissue density in the attic and mastoid highly suggestive of cholesteatoma.

followed anteriorly until the attic is opened. The superior portion of the posterior bony canal wall can be removed at this point. Cortical bone should be taken down as far as possible to the zygomatic root, and the tegmen is followed medially until the remaining portion of the scutum is identified. If the attic is filled with cholesteatoma and the scutum is partially eroded, the remaining scutum can be removed with a drill. If there is concern about injuring an intact ossicular chain, however, the scutum can be thinned down and removed with a curette.

The facial recess can be opened at this point by following the fossa incudus downward with a 2 mm diamond burr using constant suction-irrigation. Once the facial recess is opened widely, the remainder of the posterior bony canal wall can be taken down with a rongeur.

The contents of the sac are debulked, and the matrix is dissected beginning posteriorly and working forward toward

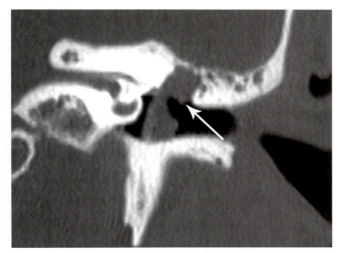

Fig. 10.7 Computed tomographic scan showing granulation tissue in the postoperative mastoid cavity (*arrow*). At surgery, there was no recurrent cholesteatoma.

the lateral semicircular canal and stapes. The lateral semicircular canal can usually be identified before removing the matrix (**Fig. 10.8B**). If fistula is suspected, the matrix should be left over the lateral canal until later in the case. If the field is infected with purulent material, it may be preferable not to remove the matrix over the lateral canal.

The incus and malleus head, if present, should be removed. The matrix is peeled away from the medial wall of the attic, working toward the tympanic segment of the facial nerve. It is wise to assume that the bony fallopian canal is dehiscent in every case. The matrix should be peeled away from the facial nerve working from above downward, avoiding sharp instruments on the nerve. The backside of a curved Rosen needle is helpful, using the tip to elevate the free edge of matrix, and sweeping the blunt surface of the instrument gently along the nerve while peeling the matrix away. The stapes should be palpated through the matrix. If the disease is adherent to the stapes, the matrix should be cut just lateral to the capitulum with a Bellucci microalligator scissors and the remainder of the disease dissected later, after better exposure is obtained.

Disease in the middle ear is dealt with as in primary surgery. The drum should be elevated first. If the middle ear space is free of disease, there may be no need to interrupt any previously made ossicular reconstruction. If on the other hand there is invagination of epithelium into the middle ear, the stapes capitulum should be separated from its attachment and the middle ear explored and all disease removed widely as in primary surgery. If the middle ear disease is extensive, it may be safer to avoid reconstruction and simply create a radical mastoidectomy cavity.

Any remaining disease must be cleared from the mastoid cavity. Once the matrix is elevated, all the remaining bony crypts need to be carefully inspected to be sure that there is no plunging disease. All remaining air cells should be exenterated with a polishing burr.

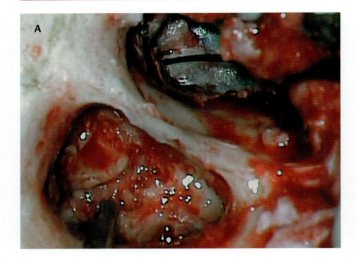

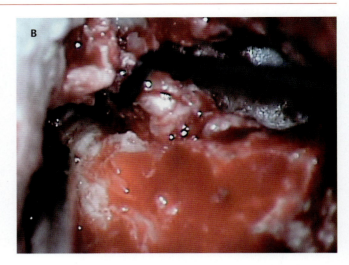

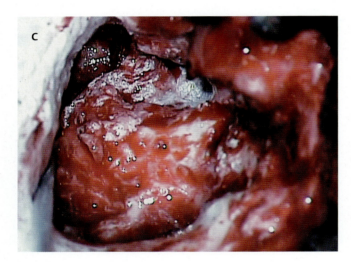

Fig. 10.8 **(A)** Recurrent cholesteatoma arising from the tympanic membrane. Gentle probing reveals extension of the disease to the attic. **(B)** After the canal wall has been taken down, the posterior limit of the sac is identified, and the matrix is elevated away from the lateral semicircular canal. **(C)** Canal wall down cavity after complete removal of recurrent disease. The bony edges have been beveled, and the facial ridge lowered to the level of the mastoid segment of the facial nerve. The cavity can be made functionally smaller by using a Palva (conchomeatal soft tissue) flap.

Cavity management is addressed after all cholesteatoma is removed. The goal is to create a compact cavity. This involves beveling all the bony edges widely, including the retrosigmoid bone (removing more bone paradoxically leads to a smaller cavity, as the soft tissues collapse medially to fill the space). The mastoid tip should be amputated down to the level of the digastric muscle. The bone anterior to the mastoid tip should be taken down so that the most dependent portion of the mastoid cavity is confluent with the inferior canal wall. In a sclerotic mastoid, the cavity can be sculpted to a round shape. In a well-pneumatized mastoid, as much cellular bone as possible should be removed. The facial ridge should be removed completely so that the facial nerve is skeletonized to a thin layer of bone (**Fig. 10.8C**), and the bone anterior to the facial nerve should be removed as well. This results in a tympanic cavity that is shallower than normal. A meatoplasty should be performed as previously described. Obliteration of the cavity with fibrous tissue flap (Palva flap) is optional in small cavities but should be performed in larger cavities, except when there is a real concern of burying residual disease.

Middle Ear Reconstruction

Ossicular reconstruction can be undertaken in revision cases, often with good results.[6] Options include the following:

- Leaving the original reconstruction intact (feasible in cases in which recurrence begins in the attic and does not involve the middle ear)
- Repairing the tympanic membrane and conducting a simultaneous ossicular repair

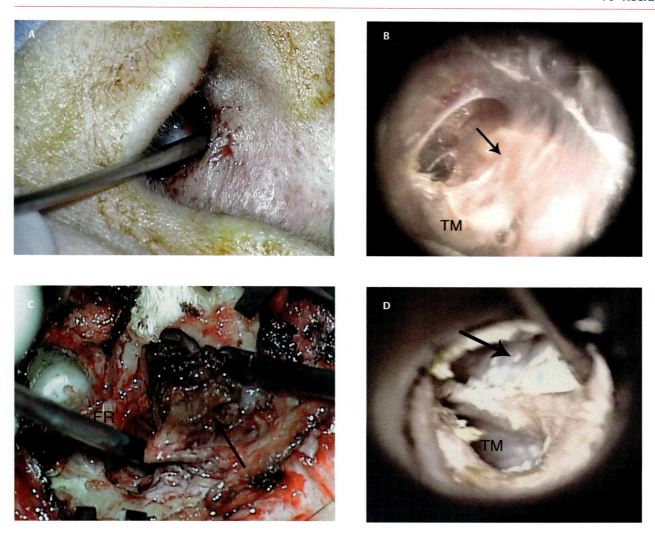

Fig. 10.9 Examples of recurrent cholesteatoma after canal wall down mastoidectomy (all left ears). **(A)** Recurrence behind meatal stenosis. **(B)** Recurrence behind membranous stenosis (*arrow*). TM, tympanic membrane. **(C)** Recurrence behind a high facial ridge (FR) (*arrow*). **(D)** Recurrence behind the membranous partition (*arrow*). TM, tympanic membrane.

- Repairing the tympanic membrane and postponing the ossicular repair
- Performing a type 4 reconstruction (cavum minor)
- Excising the drum completely and creating a radical mastoidectomy cavity

These are discussed in more detail in Chapter 3.

Revision Surgery after Canal Wall Down Mastoidectomy

Although the recurrence rate for canal wall down mastoidectomy is lower than for canal wall up, it is not zero. A well-performed canal wall down mastoidectomy should have a shallow, well-beveled cavity and an adequate meatoplasty.

Recurrence can form in the middle ear, especially in cases of posterior tympanic membrane retractions.[7] Recurrence can form behind a meatal stenosis, within a bony cavum in the mastoid tip, behind a high facial ridge, or beneath a membranous partition (**Fig. 10.9**). Recurrence can form years after the initial surgery, so patients should be encouraged to return for routine cleaning and inspection once or twice a year for life.

Recurrent cholesteatoma in a canal wall down cavity can become quite large before causing any symptoms. This will usually manifest itself as persistent infection in an existing mastoid cavity, with pain and malodorous discharge. Occasionally recurrences grow silently and are only discovered on exam. Surgical treatment consists of reexcision of the sac, with revision mastoidectomy to address any pockets of osteitis or mucosal disease, and to resculpt the cavity to

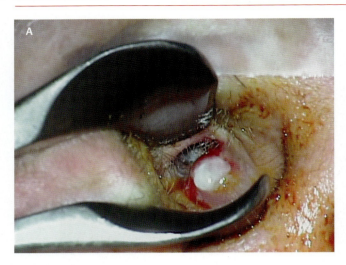
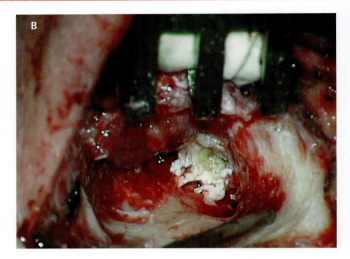

Fig. 10.10 Recurrent cholesteatoma in a left canal wall down cavity, occurring 8 years after initial procedure. **(A)** Viewed through the meatus, a large cyst can be seen, which formed subepithelially. **(B)** At surgery, this was approached via a postauricular incision. The cholesteatoma was completely excised and a meatoplasty was performed to direct the conchomeatal skin posteriorly, into the cavity.

remove any anatomical factors for further recurrence. This can be done through the meatus if the disease is well circumscribed, but a postauricular approach is usually needed for adequate exposure (**Fig. 10.10**).

Meatal stenosis can be a stubborn problem and refractory to surgical treatment. It is more common in children than adults, probably because of a more exuberant healing response. It is caused by concentric fibrosis that forms a progressively tightening scar. Failure to place periosteal stay sutures during the initial operation may be a factor. At the very least, meatal stenosis makes it difficult to clean the cavity adequately and allows squamous debris to accumulate and become secondarily infected.

An example of a meatal stenosis in a teenager with a canal wall down mastoid cavity is shown in **Fig. 10.11A**. After a lengthy trial of ototopicals, 2% acetic acid irrigations, and repeated cleanings in the office, a mutual decision was made by patient and physician to proceed with surgery. A meatoplasty was performed, first creating meatal (Lempert) incisions through skin and cartilage, then accessing the cavity through a postauricular incision (**Fig. 10.11B**). The cavity was thoroughly debrided, and a meatoplasty was completed by placing postauricular stay sutures. The meatus has remained wide, and although the cavity continues to drain, it is much easier to clean, and squamous debris has not recollected.

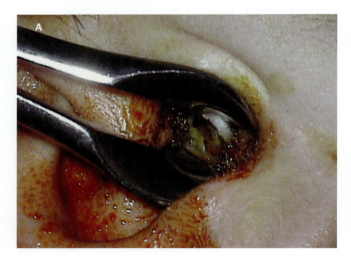
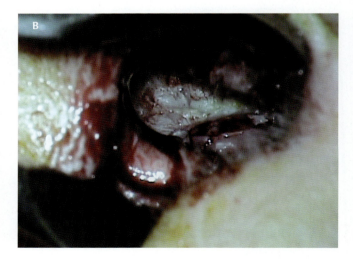

Fig. 10.11 Meatal stenosis of the right ear, causing recurrent malodorous drainage, which was difficult to clean in the office. **(A)** Small meatal opening, and infected squamous material in mastoid cavity. **(B)** At surgery, a constricted mastoid cavity without recurrent cholesteatoma. Meatoplasty was successful in creating a manageable cavity.

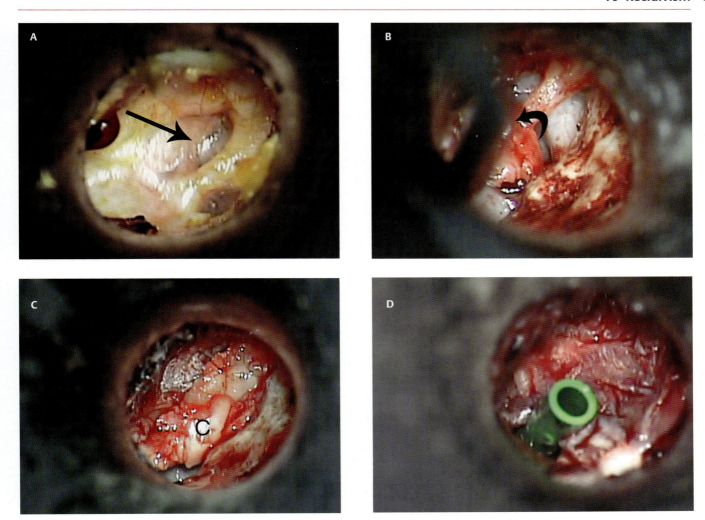

Fig. 10.12 Middle ear recurrence after canal wall up mastoidectomy, left ear. **(A)** Pars tensa retraction posterior to malleus (*arrow*). **(B)** Tympanic membrane elevated and dissected from the incus and stapes (*curved arrow*). The retraction pocket was everted and excised. **(C)** Cartilage **(C)** reconstruction of the posterior TM. **(D)** Subannular T-tube was inserted to prevent re-retraction.

Revision Tympanoplasty for Middle Ear Recurrence

In some patients with middle ear cholesteatoma, the recurrence will form in the middle ear. These cholesteatomas arise from retraction pockets in the pars tensa and grow medially toward the promontory (unlike residual cholesteatomas of the middle ear, which usually begin in the oval window or sinus tympani). These cases are best managed with excision of the sac and repair of the tympanic membrane with cartilage. The attic and mastoid do not need to be opened if the disease remains confined to the mesotympanum.

Following is a case of a 20-year-old woman with longstanding chronic ear disease and prior bilateral cholesteatoma surgery (**Fig. 10.12**). She developed progressive conductive hearing loss and retraction pocket formation on the left, enveloping the ossicles and causing early incus necrosis. She underwent tympanoplasty with cartilage graft, and placement of a T-tube. The procedure resulted in near-normal hearing, despite early incus erosion.

◆ Residual Cholesteatoma

Residual cholesteatoma is disease left behind by the surgeon. Incompletely excised cholesteatoma will regrow and eventually cause erosion or infection and lead to the same symptoms and complications as the original disease.

Residual disease in a canal wall down cavity is not an uncommon occurrence and can usually be dealt with in the office. Residual cholesteatoma appears as a well circumscribed epithelial pearl (**Fig. 10.13**). It can be excised through the meatus under the microscope. The thin mucosal lining is gently incised with the tip of a curved pick (there is little sensation) and folded open. The contents can then be shelled out with a cerumen loop. The mucosal edges should be spread apart to marsupialize the sac and prevent it from coming back.

Residual cholesteatoma is more of a problem after canal wall up mastoidectomy because it can grow to a large size before it is detected clinically. Residual cholesteatoma is the

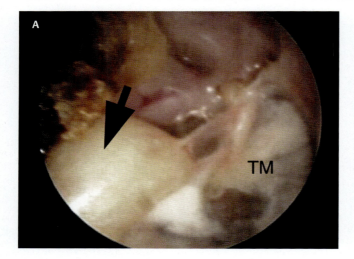
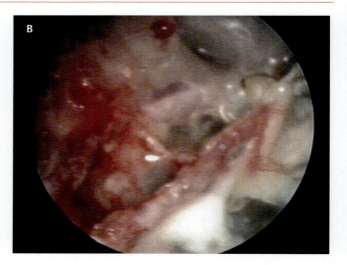

Fig. 10.13   Residual cholesteatoma in a canal wall down mastoid cavity, right ear. **(A)** The disease appears as a well circumscribed squamous pearl (*arrow*). TM, tympanic membrane. **(B)** This was excised in the office, using a sharp pick to incise the overlying mucosa and then deliver the contents.

reason that second-stage surgery is often recommended after canal wall up mastoidectomy (see Chapter 7). The chance of leaving a focus residual disease varies among different published series, but can be as high as 30%.[8] In some cases, imaging will demonstrate the residual cholesteatoma, but, as already discussed, imaging has not yet proved sensitive or specific enough to replace second-stage surgery. If left untreated, residual cholesteatoma will eventually grow and cause bone erosion through the posterior canal wall or tegmen, infection with tympanic membrane perforation or discharge, or a complication such as lateral semicircular canal fistula.

Residual cholesteatoma requires revision surgery if the disease is localized and the canal wall can be preserved, but if it is large it will usually result in canal wall down mastoidectomy. The following case illustrates this. An 11-year-old boy had a canal wall up mastoidectomy, and returned for routine follow-up, asymptomatic. A CT scan revealed a round soft tissue density in the anterior epitympanum (**Fig. 10.14A**). At surgery, a well circumscribed residual cholesteatoma was found. Because he had a large, well developed mastoid, the disease was removed by extending the transmastoid atticotomy, and the canal wall was preserved (**Fig. 10.14B**).

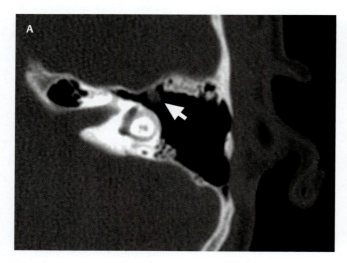
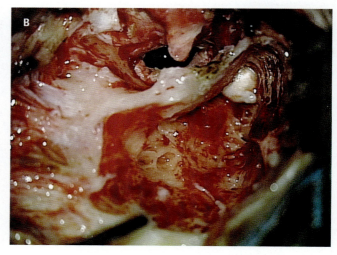

Fig. 10.14   Residual attic cholesteatoma, left ear. **(A)** Asymptomatic lesion (*arrow*) detected on computed tomographic scan. **(B)** The disease was removed via transmastoid atticotomy with endoscopic assistance, and the canal wall was preserved, avoiding a large cavity.

References

1. Yung M, Jacobsen NL, Vowler SL. A 5-year observational study of the outcome in pediatric cholesteatoma surgery. Otol Neurotol 2007;28(8): 1038–1040

2. Stankovic M. Follow-up of cholesteatoma surgery: open versus closed tympanoplasty. ORL J Otorhinolaryngol Relat Spec 2007;69(5):299–305

3. Smyth GD. Surgical treatment of cholesteatoma: the role of staging in closed operations. Ann Otol Rhinol Laryngol 1988;97(6 Pt 1):667–669

4. Jeunen G, Desloovere C, Hermans R, Vandecaveye V. The value of magnetic resonance imaging in the diagnosis of residual or recurrent acquired cholesteatoma after canal wall-up tympanoplasty. Otol Neurotol 2008;29(1):16–18

5. De Foer B, Vercruysse JP, Bernaerts A, et al. Detection of postoperative residual cholesteatoma with non-echo-planar diffusion-weighted magnetic resonance imaging. Otol Neurotol 2008;29(4):513–517

6. Kaylie DM, Gardner EK, Jackson CG. Revision chronic ear surgery. Otolaryngol Head Neck Surg 2006;134(3):443–450

7. Ajalloueyan M. Experience with surgical management of cholesteatomas. Arch Otolaryngol Head Neck Surg 2006;132(9):931–933

8. Sheehy JL, Brackmann DE, Graham MD. Cholesteatoma surgery: residual and recurrent disease: a review of 1,024 cases. Ann Otol Rhinol Laryngol 1977;86(4 Pt 1):451–462

11

Complications of the Disease

Acute and chronic otitis media, with or without cholesteatoma, consists of inflammation of the pneumatized spaces of the temporal bone, which include the eustachian tube, middle ear, and mastoid air cell system. By convention, the definition of a *complication* of otitis media is the spread of infection outside the temporal bone. The most commonly used classification includes *intratemporal* (or "aural") and *intracranial* complications (**Table 11.1**). Intratemporal complications include mastoiditis, labyrinthitis, facial paralysis, and petrositis. Intracranial complications include meningitis, brain abscess, epidural abscess, subdural abscess, sigmoid (or lateral) sinus thrombosis, and otitic hydrocephalus.

It is commonly understood that complications of otitis media have become quite rare since the advent of antibiotics. However, because of their low incidence, complications are sometimes overlooked, or their diagnosis is delayed because of lack of recognition. For example, children with facial paralysis secondary to otitis media are sometimes mistakenly treated for Bell palsy, without attention given to treating the middle ear suppuration. It is therefore imperative that otologists who treat inflammatory middle ear disease be familiar with all the complications and their proper management. Many of the complications of otitis media nowadays are seen in poorer urban centers,[1] or in immigrants from developing countries.

Table 11.1 Complications of Otitis Media (with or without Cholesteatoma)

Aural Complications	Intracranial Complications
Mastoiditis	Meningitis
Labyrinthitis	Epidural abscess
Facial paralysis	Subdural abscess
Petrositis	Brain abscess
	Sigmoid sinus thrombosis
	Otitic hydrocephalus

◆ Mastoiditis

Mastoiditis occurs when there is coalescence of mastoid air cells. Mastoiditis is the process of liquefactive necrosis of bone. It can occur after acute or chronic otitis media, but the chronic form usually involves cholesteatoma. Otitis media is a suppurative infection of the middle ear. It passes through stages of hyperemia, exudation, suppuration, and (usually) resolution. In the rare event that the suppurative process does not resolve, liquefactive necrosis of bone can occur and an abscess can form. In the most common scenario, the pus erodes the mastoid cortex near the MacEwan triangle and forms a subperiosteal abscess; rarely it can erode through other weak points in the temporal bone—anteriorly at the zygomatic root, or inferiorly through the digastric ridge into the deep spaces of the neck (Bezold abscess).[2]

Cholesteatoma permits the formation of coalescent mastoiditis by blocking the egress of pus from the mastoid into the middle ear. The so-called attic-antral block causes pus to accumulate in the mastoid under pressure and erode the cortical bone to escape into the subperiosteal or neck spaces. Acute mastoiditis associated with cholesteatoma is relatively rare, occurring in approximately one of 40 cases of mastoiditis.[3]

Acute mastoiditis presents in an acutely ill patient, often with fever and systemic signs. Mastoiditis that develops after acute otitis media classically occurs 2 weeks after the acute infection, but mastoiditis that develops from chronic suppurative otitis media can occur at any time in the course of the disease.[4] The clinical signs of a subperiosteal abscess include a tender, fluctuant swelling in the postauricular sulcus, protrusion of the auricle, and "sagging" of the posterior canal wall (**Fig. 11.1**). A Bezold abscess, less commonly seen, presents with tenderness, redness, swelling, and stiffness of the neck (**Fig. 11.2**).

The radiologic hallmark of mastoiditis is coalescence, or loss of the bony septations of the mastoid (*N.B.:* radiologists will often read opacification of the mastoid air cells as "mastoiditis"; while this is technically correct in the radiologic sense, acute or serous otitis media routinely causes diffuse

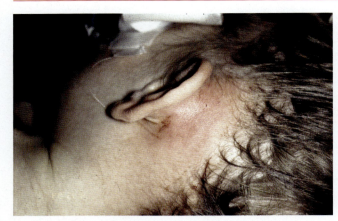

Fig. 11.1 Acute coalescent mastoiditis, left ear, causing a subperiosteal abscess with auricular protrusion, posterior canal wall sagging, and a red, tender postauricular swelling, in an infant.

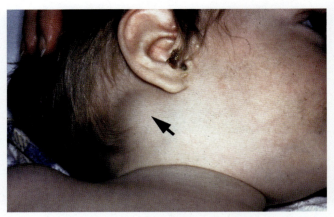

Fig. 11.2 A Bezold abscess of the right neck (*arrow*) occurring after acute coalescent mastoiditis. The suppuration spreads form the mastoid to the deep spaces of the neck via a break in the digastric ridge.

opacification of the mastoid air cells, and this is not equivalent to "mastoiditis" in the clinical sense). Plain films of the mastoid will demonstrate coalescence, but these have become scarcer as computed tomographic (CT) scanners have become ubiquitous. On CT, coalescence will appear as loss of bony septations (not different in appearance from any cholesteatoma); the abscess will appear as a dome-shaped fluid collection in the subperiosteal space, accompanied by a focal interruption of the bony cortex (**Fig. 11.3**).

The bacteriology of acute mastoiditis usually consists of pyogenic organisms, of which *Streptococcus pneumoniae* is most common. Chronic suppurative otitis media is more likely to be caused by *Pseudomonas* sp., other gram-negative rods. *Staphylococcus aureus* is also occasionally seen, and methicillin-resistant *S. aureus* (MRSA) is increasing in prevalence and can be difficult to eradicate.

Treatment of mastoiditis consists of culture of the ear canal drainage, intravenous fluids and antibiotics, and urgent surgery to drain the abscess and remove its source. The surgical

drainage of a subperiosteal abscess is performed through a postauricular incision (**Fig. 11.4**). The periosteum is usually very thick and edematous, and tented by the abscess. A stab incision of the periosteum usually releases pus under pressure, and the fluid should be evacuated and cultured, and the wound irrigated thoroughly. The periosteal incision is lengthened, and the mastoid cortex exposed. The cortex can be opened with a cutting burr. There may be more bleeding than usual, so constant suction-irrigation is advisable. The mastoidectomy is then completed and the cholesteatoma removed. If there is too much inflammation to do this safely, then after the mastoid is decorticated, the wound can be closed loosely over a Penrose drain and the completion mastoidectomy postponed for a week or two until the inflammation subsides.

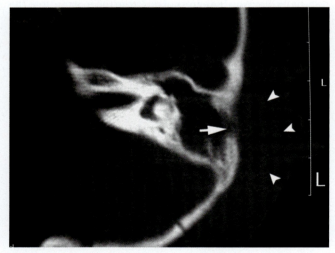

Fig. 11.3 Computed tomographic appearance of acute coalescent mastoiditis, axial view, left ear. Coalescence appears as a loss of bony septations; the abscess is a dome-shaped fluid collection in the subperiosteal space (*arrowheads*), accompanied by a focal interruption of the bony cortex (*arrow*).

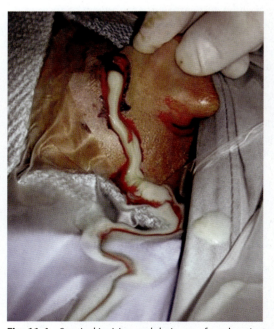

Fig. 11.4 Surgical incision and drainage of a subperiosteal abscess, left ear. After the thick periosteal rind is incised, pus comes forth under pressure. The material should be cultured, and the abscess cavity evacuated and copiously irrigated.

Recent attention has been given to the nonsurgical management of acute mastoiditis, but this remains a matter of controversy.[5] It is not clear that all these cases meet the criteria for acute mastoiditis—some cases of postauricular swelling may reflect periosteitis rather than a florid abscess. In any case, if cholesteatoma is present, surgical therapy is not optional and should be instituted as soon as the patient is stable to undergo the procedure.

◆ Labyrinthitis

Labyrinthitis is extension of inflammation to the inner ear and manifests clinically as sensorineural hearing loss and vestibular impairment. According to Schuknecht,[6] infectious labyrinthitis can be toxic or suppurative. Toxic, or serous, labyrinthitis is caused by bacterial toxins that enter the fluids of the inner ear. The portal of entry may be the round or oval window membrane, or through an acquired fistula. The degree of cochlear and vestibular impairment is variable, as is the degree of recovery. Milder cases are characterized pathologically by endolymphatic hydrops and proteinaceous precipitates in the endolymph; more severe cases have degeneration of the sense organs, and so loss of cochlear and vestibular function may be permanent. Sometimes toxic labyrinthitis is diagnosed retrospectively, when sensorineural hearing loss occurs in the setting of chronic ear disease.

Suppurative labyrinthitis is characterized by polymorphonuclear cells in the perilymph and later in the endolymph. Necrosis of the membranous labyrinth can ensue, and the infection can spread intracranially. Fibrous, and later bony, obliteration of the labyrinth (*labyrinthitis ossificans*) can occur over time.

Chronic labyrinthitis is characterized by progressive destruction of the bony labyrinth, endolymphatic hydrops, proteinaceous exudates, and later degeneration of the sense organs and labyrinthine sclerosis.

Labyrinthine fistula can be caused by cholesteatoma and can be the portal of infection into the labyrinth (see Chapter 6).

Sensorineural hearing loss can be a late manifestation of chronic labyrinthitis in the presence of cholesteatoma. Sensorineural hearing loss has been found to occur with higher incidence in chronic otitis media than in the general population.[7,8]

◆ Facial Nerve Paralysis

The facial nerve is a hearty nerve with a myelin sheath, and so paresis caused by infection is not common. The facial nerve is protected by a bony shell in the middle ear. Natural dehiscences occur in at least 8% of cases,[9] but the incidence is higher in the presence of cholesteatoma.[10–12] Paresis of immediate onset usually signifies suppuration against a bare nerve. Paresis of gradual onset is the result of pressure against the nerve, usually by cholesteatoma.

The first circumstance requires urgent surgery—the goal should be to drain the pus. If the eardrum is intact and the patient has acute otitis media, a wide myringotomy should be performed and the middle ear fluid should be cultured and antibiotics started. This condition has a good prognosis provided the treatment is done as soon as possible after the onset of the problem.[13] Myringotomy is usually sufficient treatment, unless the facial paralysis occurs in the setting of acute mastoiditis (bony coalescence with subperiosteal abscess); in this situation, mastoidectomy will be necessary to provide adequate surgical drainage.

On the other hand, when the onset of facial paresis is gradual, or if facial paralysis occurs in the setting of chronic suppurative otitis media, the prognosis is not as good. In these cases, surgery is indicated, with the goal of removing the infected focus from against the nerve (ie, to perform a tympanomastoidectomy to remove the cholesteatoma). In this event, the prognosis for recovery of facial nerve function is variable and depends on the length of time the paresis has been present before surgery. Paralysis that is present for 1 week or less usually recovers;[14] paralysis of greater than 1 year does not.[13] Paresis that develops slowly will usually take weeks to recover. If the paresis is long-standing, fibrosis will develop that will prevent the nerve from recovering completely.

Three cases are presented to illustrate these principles. In the first, a small child came to the emergency room with earache and fever and facial paralysis of acute onset. Examination revealed a red, bulging tympanic membrane. In a crying child, it is relatively easy to assess the status of the facial nerve (**Fig. 11.5**). He was started on antibiotics and a wide myringotomy was performed to evacuate pus from the middle ear. The infection resolved and the facial paralysis recovered fully within a few days.

The second case is an elderly woman who presented with gradual onset facial paralysis. She had a history of mastoid surgery in that ear 20 years earlier, but the details were not known. Examination revealed complete (grade VI) facial pa-

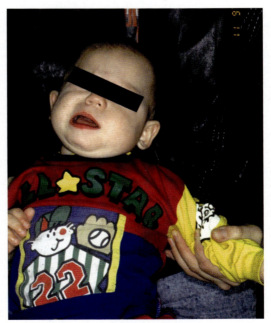

Fig. 11.5 Acute facial paralysis, left side, as a complication of acute otitis media in a child.

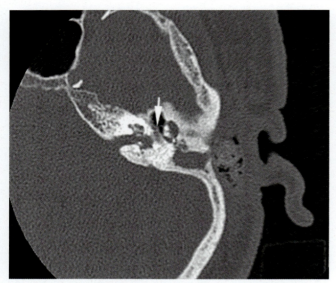

Fig. 11.6 Axial computed tomographic scan of a cholesteatoma of the left ear causing acute facial paralysis. The facial nerve is visible (*arrow*).

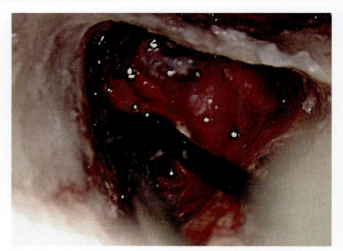

Fig. 11.7 Dissection of granulation tissue off the facial nerve, right ear.

ralysis and drainage from the ear (**Fig. 11.6**). At surgery, a small pars tensa cholesteatoma was discovered medial to the incus and pressing against an exposed tympanic segment of the facial nerve. A canal wall down mastoidectomy was performed with removal of the incus along with the disease. The ear healed well and the facial nerve recovered completely within 3 months.

The third case is a 50-year-old man with chronic ear drainage and facial paralysis of gradual onset over 1 or 2 weeks. He had a radical mastoid cavity in his other ear for a history of cholesteatoma. At surgery, there was a tympanic membrane perforation and abundant granulation tissue with pus in the middle ear and mastoid. A canal wall up mastoidectomy with facial recess was performed, and the granulation tissue was completely removed, dissecting it off the exposed facial nerve (**Fig. 11.7**). Cultures showed *S. aureus*, and the patient was treated with ciprofloxacin orally and ofloxacin drops postoperatively. The paralysis recovered completely over a 3-week period. However, the ear drainage later recurred and the hearing did not improve.

◆ Petrositis

This rare complication occurs when the petrous apex air cells become infected, causing a triad of symptoms, termed Gradenigo syndrome, consisting of purulent ear discharge, retrobulbar pain (from trigeminal nerve irritation), and lateral rectus palsy (caused by sixth nerve involvement in the Dorello canal). The petrous apex cells are often pneumatized, and suppurative infection can become trapped there if there is outflow obstruction to the middle ear (**Fig. 11.8**). This situation might occur in the presence of giant cholesteatoma ("petrous temporal bone cholesteatoma"), or in cholesteatosis where the extensive disease involves the petrous apex cells (see Chapter 6). The treatment consists of surgical evacuation of the cholesteatoma from all the involved areas.

The petrous apex is relatively difficult to approach surgically; this area communicates with the mastoid through infralabyrinthine, retrolabyrinthine, and supralabyrinthine cell tracts. The bony pathway created by the erosive disease will usually provide surgical access; in very advanced cases, a labyrinthectomy might be necessary to evacuate all the disease.[15]

Primary cholesteatomas of the petrous apex can also occur.[16] These are actually *epidermoid tumors* and are not related pathogenetically to the acquired cholesteatomas that are the principal subject of this book. These uncommon tumors appear radiologically as solid tumors of the petrous apex. They can present with any of the features of petrous apicitis, or with an intracranial mass effect, or as an incidental radiographic finding. On CT they appear as expansile lesions that erode the bony cortex. On magnetic resonance imaging (MRI), they have imaging characteristics that follow cerebrospinal fluid (CSF); they are hypodense on T1-weighted

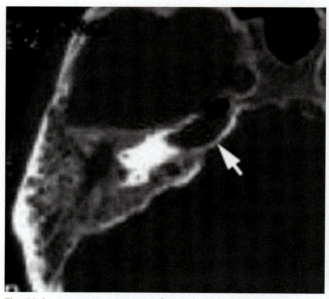

Fig. 11.8 Acute petrositis, opacification and air-fluid level of the right petrous apex (*arrow*).

images, hyperintense on T2, and do not enhance with gadolinium. Surgical access can be gained through a transcochlear, posterior fossa or middle cranial fossa approach. These lesions are difficult to eradicate and readily regrow if they are not completely resected.

◆ Intracranial Complications

Intracranial spread of infection from the mastoid can cause meningitis, brain abscess, epidural abscess, or subdural empyema. Spread of infection to the sigmoid sinus can cause septic thrombophlebitis of that structure ("lateral sinus thrombosis"), in addition to intracranial infection. Venous thrombosis may also result in increased intracranial pressure, or "otitic hydrocephalus." Intracranial complications often may cause headache or fever without focal neurological signs. Although CT scanning is instrumental in determining the extent of disease in the mastoid, MRI is most useful in demonstrating intracranial complications.[17]

Meningitis can be otogenic in origin, occurring more commonly with acute otitis media than with chronic otitis or cholesteatoma,[18] but it is not always clear that the middle ear process is causal.[19] Infection can spread intracranially through bony channels or hematogenously.[20] The diagnosis is made by lumbar puncture; CSF culture and sensitivity are mandatory, and treatment is by immediate administration of intravenous antibiotics. *Pneumococcus* has surpassed *Haemophilus* as the most common organism.[18] Bedside myringotomy can be performed adjunctively if there is a bulging tympanic membrane, but if mastoiditis is present this should be treated by urgent mastoidectomy.[20] Meningitis can lead to permanent sensorineural hearing loss and cochlear ossification, so steroid administration is recommended, especially in children.

Brain abscess classically presents with focal neurological signs or seizures, but nowadays the majority cause only headache or fever and the abscess is discovered on CT scan[21] (**Fig. 11.9**). Otogenic brain abscesses occur either in the cerebellum or in the temporal lobe and develop by either hematogenous or contiguous spread. Neurosurgical consultation should be routinely sought. The treatment of the abscess consists of prolonged medical treatment with culture-appropriate antibiotics, in addition to single or repeated aspiration, or occasionally excision of the lesion.[22] The ear pathology can be addressed surgically when the patient's neurological status is stabilized. Needle aspiration can occasionally be performed through the mastoidectomy.[23] Small abscesses may be treated with antibiotics alone. *Streptococcus* sp., anaerobes, and *Enterobacter* are the most commonly isolated organisms.[21,24] Interestingly the ear and abscess cultures do not always concur.[21]

Epidural abscess occurs when there is erosion of the tegmen or posterior fossa bony plate by disease in the mastoid. Epidural granulation tissue is a fairly common finding during mastoidectomy for chronic ear disease, but a true collection of pus in the epidural space is relatively rare. Epidural abscess appears to be more common than brain abscess in the pediatric age group.[15] The patient will have headache, fever, and focal meningeal signs. MRI will demonstrate the abscess (**Fig. 11.10A**),[17] and CT will show the site of bony erosion (**Fig. 11.10B**). The abscess can be evacuated through a transmastoid approach by removing the overlying bone.

Lateral sinus thrombosis is a rare complication in which a septic thrombus forms in the lateral venous (sigmoid) sinus. The incidence has become very low in the antibiotic era, and the clinical presentation has changed. The classically described syndrome of headache, otorrhea, and spiking ("picket fence") fevers is not often seen; instead patients are likely to present with headache and neurological findings including VI or VII nerve palsies or signs of increased intracranial pressure, without fever or ear complaints.[25] Lateral sinus thrombosis can be seen in the clinical context of acute otitis media, with or without mastoiditis, or chronic otitis media, with or without cholesteatoma.

Imaging studies are helpful and may have eliminated the need for needle aspiration of the sinus in making the diagnosis.[26] CT of the temporal bones with contrast will demonstrate enhancement of the soft tissues around the sinus and a filling void within the lumen, termed a delta sign (**Fig. 11.11A**).[27] MRI will display increased signal intensities on T1- and T2-weighted images indicating venous stasis (**Fig. 11.11B**), and gadolinium-enhanced MRI may outline the thrombus. Magnetic resonance venography will demonstrate the absence of flow. Doppler ultrasonography can demonstrate occlusion of the lateral sinus or extension of a thrombus along the internal jugular vein. MRI will also demonstrate any concurrent intracranial pathology; in one series, brain abscess, epidural abscess, and subperiosteal abscess were found to coexist in patients with lateral sinus thrombosis.[26]

Lateral sinus thrombosis should be regarded as a grave complication, and immediate treatment should be initiated with hospitalization and intravenous antibiotics. Mastoidectomy should be performed and the sigmoid sinus unroofed. Classically, the sinus is aspirated with a 25 gauge needle, and if no blood or pus is retrieved, the sinus is filleted open and the septic clot evacuated. Venous backbleeding can be

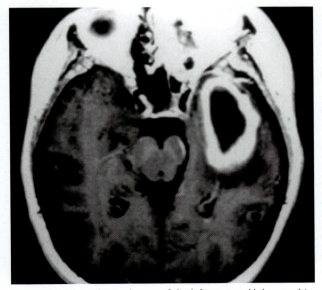

Fig. 11.9 A large brain abscess of the left temporal lobe, resulting from chronic otitis media.

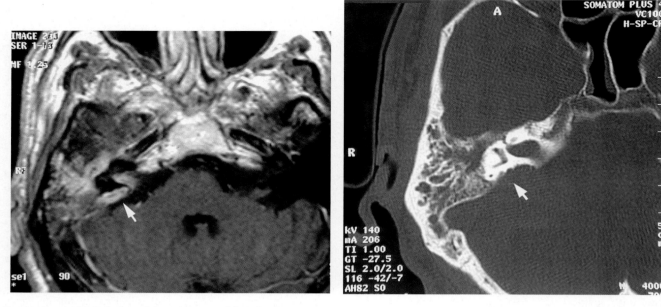

Fig. 11.10 Epidural abscess of the right mastoid. **(A)** The abscess is located near the endolymphatic sac and has eroded the adjacent otic capsule bone (*arrow*). **(B)** Magnetic resonance imaging demonstrates contrast enhancement of the corresponding area (*arrow*).

controlled with extraluminal packing with oxidized cellulose or sclerosants.[28] Syms et al have recently advocated nonsurgical management of the thrombosed sinus, contending that with intravenous antibiotics and low-dose heparin the sinus will eventually recanalize.[26] Conservative management of the sinus was also successful in other series.[25,27] Manolidis and Kutz, on the other hand, have argued that because of the increased prevalence of antibiotic resistance, evacuation of the thrombosed sinus is essential.[28] The use of anticoagulation

is controversial, but it is probably warranted if thrombosis extends to the torcula, because thrombosis of the superior sagittal sinus is a grave complication.

Otitic hydrocephalus is a rare and poorly understood condition, characterized by signs of increased intracranial pressure (headache, nausea, papilledema), usually developing insidiously.[29] Occasionally the cause will be lateral sinus thrombosis, as proven by CT/MRI, and this should be treated accordingly. In other cases, the otogenic source will be in question. Otitic

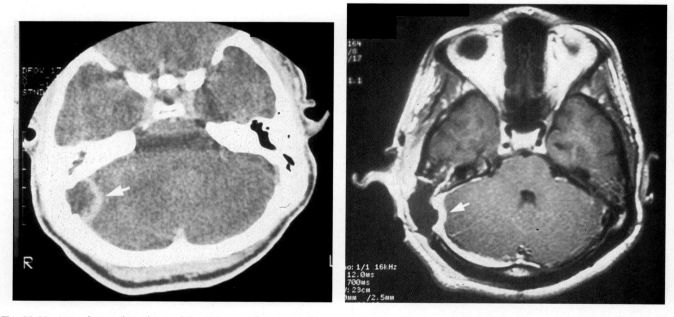

Fig. 11.11 Lateral sinus thrombosis of the right ear. **(A)** Computed tomography shows thrombosis and mural enhancement of the right sigmoid sinus (*arrow*), and opacification of the mastoid air cells. **(B)** Magnetic resonance imaging shows venous stasis of the sigmoid and transverse sinuses (*arrow*).

hydrocephalus is treated with steroids, acetazolamide, and sometimes serial lumbar puncture for CSF drainage.

◆ Conclusion

Complications of otitis media and cholesteatoma have become rare but continue to occur sporadically and must be recognized and treated promptly and aggressively. Mastoiditis occurs when there is bony coalescence; though early cases might successfully be treated with antibiotics alone, the presence of a subperiosteal abscess almost always necessitates surgery, and cholesteatoma when present must always be removed. Labyrinthitis can take on different degrees of aggressiveness; permanent loss of sensorineural and vestibular function often results despite treatment. Facial nerve paralysis requires wide myringotomy in the setting of purulent otitis media, and surgical mastoidectomy with nerve exploration when cholesteatoma is present, in addition to antibiotics and steroids. Petrositis is rare and demands surgical drainage, with the route selected according to the patient's anatomy. Intracranial complications are grave and require aggressive medical treatment. Surgical drainage is needed for lateral sinus thrombosis and epidural abscess, and for removal of cholesteatoma. Brain abscess requires neurosurgical consultation; these are treated with repeated aspiration, or nonoperatively in selected cases.

References

1. Greenberg JS, Manolidis S. High incidence of complications encountered in chronic otitis media surgery in a U.S. metropolitan public hospital. Otolaryngol Head Neck Surg 2001;125(6):623–627
2. Smouha EE, Levenson MJ, Anand VK, Parisier SC. Modern presentations of Bezold's abscess. Arch Otolaryngol Head Neck Surg 1989;115(9):1126–1129
3. Shaffer HL, Gates GA, Meyerhoff WL. Acute mastoiditis and cholesteatoma. Otolaryngology 1978;86(3 Pt 1):ORL394–ORL399
4. van den Aardweg MTA, Rovers MM, de Ru JA, Albers FW, Schilder AG. A systematic review of diagnostic criteria for acute mastoiditis in children. Otol Neurotol 2008;29(6):751–757
5. Niv A, Nash M, Peiser J, et al. Outpatient management of acute mastoiditis with periosteitis in children. Int J Pediatr Otorhinolaryngol 1998;46(1-2):9–13
6. Schuknecht HF. Pathology of the Ear. 2nd ed. Malverne, PA: Lea and Febiger; 1993:211–217
7. da Costa SS, Rosito LP, Dornelles C. Sensorineural hearing loss in patients with chronic otitis media. Eur Arch Otorhinolaryngol 2009;266(2):221–224
8. Eisenman DJ, Parisier SC. Is chronic otitis media with cholesteatoma associated with neurosensory hearing loss? Am J Otol 1998;19(1):20–25
9. Bayazit YA, Ozer E, Kanlikama M. Gross dehiscence of the bone covering the facial nerve in the light of otological surgery. J Laryngol Otol 2002;116(10):800–803
10. Moody MW, Lambert PR. Incidence of dehiscence of the facial nerve in 416 cases of cholesteatoma. Otol Neurotol 2007;28(3):400–404
11. Lin JC, Ho KY, Kuo WR, Wang LF, Chai CY, Tsai SM. Incidence of dehiscence of the facial nerve at surgery for middle ear cholesteatoma. Otolaryngol Head Neck Surg 2004;131(4):452–456
12. Selesnick SH, Lynn-Macrae AG. The incidence of facial nerve dehiscence at surgery for cholesteatoma. Otol Neurotol 2001;22(2):129–132
13. Makeham TP, Croxson GR, Coulson S. Infective causes of facial nerve paralysis. Otol Neurotol 2007;28(1):100–103
14. Quaranta N, Cassano M, Quaranta A. Facial paralysis associated with cholesteatoma: a review of 13 cases. Otol Neurotol 2007;28(3):405–407
15. Isaacson B, Kutz JW, Roland PS. Lesions of the petrous apex: diagnosis and management. Otolaryngol Clin North Am 2007;40(3):479–519, viii
16. Muckle RP, De la Cruz A, Lo WM. Petrous apex lesions. Am J Otol 1998;19(2):219–225
17. Dobben GD, Raofi B, Mafee MF, Kamel A, Mercurio S. Otogenic intracranial inflammations: role of magnetic resonance imaging. Top Magn Reson Imaging 2000;11(2):76–86
18. Migirov L, Duvdevani S, Kronenberg J. Otogenic intracranial complications: a review of 28 cases. Acta Otolaryngol 2005;125(8):819–822
19. Smith JA, Danner CJ. Complications of chronic otitis media and cholesteatoma. Otolaryngol Clin North Am 2006;39(6):1237–1255
20. Dubey SP, Larawin V, Molumi CP. Intracranial spread of chronic middle ear suppuration. Am J Otolaryngol 2010;31(2):73–77
21. Couloigner V, Sterkers O, Redondo A, Rey A. Brain abscesses of ear, nose, and throat origin: comparison between otogenic and sinogenic etiologies. Skull Base Surg 1998;8(4):163–168
22. Isaacson B, Mirabal C, Kutz JW Jr, Lee KH, Roland PS. Pediatric otogenic intracranial abscesses. Otolaryngol Head Neck Surg 2010;142(3):434–437
23. Wanna GB, Dharamsi LM, Moss JR, Bennett ML, Thompson RC, Haynes DS. Contemporary management of intracranial complications of otitis media. Otol Neurotol 2010;31(1):111–117
24. Tandon S, Beasley N, Swift AC. Changing trends in intracranial abscesses secondary to ear and sinus disease. J Laryngol Otol 2009;123(3):283–288
25. Bales CB, Sobol S, Wetmore R, Elden LM. Lateral sinus thrombosis as a complication of otitis media: 10-year experience at the children's hospital of Philadelphia. Pediatrics 2009;123(2):709–713
26. Syms MJ, Tsai PD, Holtel MR. Management of lateral sinus thrombosis. Laryngoscope 1999;109(10):1616–1620
27. Kutluhan A, Kiriş M, Yurttaş V, Kiroğlu AF, Unal O. When can lateral sinus thrombosis be treated conservatively? J Otolaryngol 2004;33(2):107–110
28. Manolidis SJ, Kutz JW Jr. Diagnosis and management of lateral sinus thrombosis. Otol Neurotol 2005;26(5):1045–1051
29. Kuczkowski J, Dubaniewicz-Wybieralska M, Przewoźny T, Narozny W, Mikaszewski B. Otitic hydrocephalus associated with lateral sinus thrombosis and acute mastoiditis in children. Int J Pediatr Otorhinolaryngol 2006;70(10):1817–1823

12

Complications of the Surgery

The complications of cholesteatoma surgery relate to recurrence, residual, or recidivism of the disease, infection, cavity management, and loss of the specialized functions of the ear.

◆ Recurrence, Residual, Recidivism

Recurrence, residual, and recidivism are known complications of cholesteatoma surgery and are discussed in detail in Chapter 8. The frequency of these is somewhat dependent on the severity of the disease (cholesteatoma and infection) at the time of surgery. Recidivism is not always considered a surgical complication because it results from the aggressive nature of the disease, but it can be prevented (or its incidence lessened) by good surgical technique, so the surgeon should regard its occurrence as a complication of form.

◆ Infection

Postoperative infection may be a complication of surgery as in surgical procedures for other diseases, or because of the inherent nature of cholesteatoma, where infection is often present at the time of surgery, even in the absence of suppuration. Cholesteatoma harbors bacteria and often presents with purulent discharge. Despite the wish to operate on the ear while it is dry, it is sometimes necessary to remove the disease to bring the infection under control, and it is also possible to develop postoperative infection from dormant bacteria in the lesion. Chronic otitis media without cholesteatoma is likewise associated with chronic mucositis, osteitis, and perforation that allows for outside contamination. Postoperative infection manifests itself as pain, swelling of the auricle or the postauricular wound, purulent discharge, and occasionally fever. Sometimes the infection is not obvious until the packing is removed 1 week postop when pus underneath the packing and a fetid odor are noted. Once discovered, culture and Gram stain should be taken, all nonresorbable pack-

ing removed, and the patient started on oral antibiotics and drops. Gram-negative organisms (*Pseudomonas*, *Proteus*, *Escherichia coli*) and *Staphylococcus aureus* (sometimes methicillin resistant) are most common. Ciprofloxacin is a good initial choice of drug until cultures return.

The chronic draining cavity can be a problem after canal wall down mastoidectomy. This may be caused by persistent granulation tissue, either along the lines of the meatal incisions, where new skin has failed to heal in, or at the base of the cavity, where persistent mastoid cells remain filled with mucosa rather than squamous epithelium. Treatment of the draining ear is by suctioning or swabbing wet material in the office setting (sometimes indecorously referred to as "toilet"), debriding any accumulated cerumen and squamous debris, and applying topical agents. A variety of medicaments have been devised for this purpose, but boric acid powder, applied through an atomizer, seems to work well as a bactericidal and drying agent. Other agents include wet or dry Gentian violet, a combination of antimicrobial agents in powder form such as CSTF (chloramphenicol, sulfa, tolnaftate, and Fungizone [Bristol-Myers Squibb, New York, NY]) powder, or 3% acetic acid drops. Acidification of the ear is initially attempted and then the antimicrobial agents are utilized if acidification does not reverse the process. Patches of granulation tissue can be lightly cauterized with silver nitrate (for larger areas) or 50% trichloroacetic acid (TCA). Care should be taken not to apply cauterizing agents to an exposed facial nerve. The draining ear may require frequent office visits at first, but the condition usually settles down over time in the majority of cases.[1]

Occasionally, the draining cavity can become refractory despite these measures, and revision surgery can be considered. The aim in these cases is to remove pockets of infected tissue, remove retained secreting air cells, lowering the posterior canal wall, removal of superior bony canal wall to the non-aircell tegmen, to provide drainage and aeration of the cavity and provide an adequate conchomeatoplasty to prevent retention of disease.[2] A computed tomographic (CT) scan may be useful if focal osteitis is suspected. Sometimes a recurrent cholesteatoma may be discovered only during

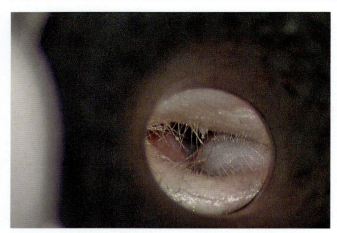

Fig. 12.1 A blue-domed cyst of the mastoid cavity (cholesterol granuloma).

revision surgery because occasionally epithelial healing of the cavity will close over deep retraction areas, especially surrounding the otic capsule (superior to the superior semicircular canal or posterior semicircular canal). Revision surgery should address each of these elements. The principles should be followed as in primary canal wall down surgery (as outlined in Chapter 4, Creating a Manageable Cavity), namely, creating a round, shallow cavity with beveled edges, lowering the facial ridge, eliminating the mastoid tip, and creating a wide meatus. The latter cannot be overemphasized—a generous meatoplasty including removal of much of the conchal and occasional antihelical cartilage is important to long-term success. In addition, all cellular bone should be exenterated, and the depth of cavity polished with a coarse diamond burr. Sometimes a split-thickness skin graft is useful to resurface the floor of the cavity,[3] but we have not often found this to be necessary.

Cholesterol granuloma cysts are blue-domed mucosal cysts that form in the floor of the antrum or in the sinodural angle. If they are asymptomatic, these can simply be followed. Occasionally, though, they cause discharge or pain and should be removed. Usually they can be incised, evacuated, and marsupialized in an office setting, but they do tend to re-collect (**Fig. 12.1**).

◆ Meatal Stenosis

Meatal stenosis is usually an error of technique. The meatoplasty is an important step in canal wall down surgery. The technique of meatoplasty was reviewed in Chapter 5. The success of meatoplasty depends upon resecting (or at least breaking the spring of) the conchal cartilage, lengthening the canal incisions to create a conchomeatal flap, and using stay sutures to ensure meatal patency.[4] When restenosis occurs, the meatoplasty might need to be revised. In these cases, a postauricular approach should be used, a strip of conchal cartilage is taken, and stay sutures should be placed between the subcutaneous tissue of the conchomeatal flap and the perichondrium of the concha. These sutures are important for keeping the meatus open. Nonresorbable packing

should also be placed but should not be relied upon. Long-term stents can be used in stubborn cases.

In canal wall up surgery, a posterior and superior bony canalplasty is often performed to better visualize the disease process. In these patients it is helpful to perform a limited meatoplasty by making an extended superior soft tissue canal incision and removing soft tissue and sometimes a rim of superior conchal cartilage. The intraoperative packing is important to maintain this opening, and Silastic sheeting may be used against the bone with interior packing. Reapproximating the periosteal incisions at the end of the procedure is also important to prevent meatal collapse.

◆ Medial Stenosis

Medial stenosis can also occur. In canal wall up surgery, this is caused by subcutaneous fibrosis of distal canal skin, or by adhesions from the posterior canal skin to the anterior canal wall, or to "blunting" of the tympanic membrane in the anterior sulcus. Stenosis can be prevented by carefully redraping the skin flaps at the end of the surgical procedure, and by using nonadherent packing in the canal lumen. *Blunting* is a special and frequent problem that comes about when an overlay graft technique is used,[5] or when the anterior rim of the tympanic membrane is lacking and the tympanic membrane graft is allowed to ride up the anterior bony canal. Carefully and accurately placing the graft under the anterior bony annulus may help prevent this. Once blunting has occurred, it will usually resist attempts at correction by revision surgery. Correction of blunting requires revision of the tympanoplasty by an experienced surgeon. After the anterior canal skin is incised and elevated, a fascial graft should be placed medial to the bony annulus of the ear canal, and a sliding graft of canal skin or partial-thickness skin graft is used to reconstruct the anterior and superior canal wall skin.[6] Packing is important in these cases, and it is preferable to use Silastic sheeting followed by careful internal packing.

Medial stenosis can also occur after canal wall down surgery. This usually takes the form of a membranous partition that forms across the attic or antrum. At times this is a useful development in that it limits the functional size of the cavity (by acting as a "soft wall" reconstruction), but it does create a potential space for recurrent disease to form that cannot be accessed through the meatus (an example of this is illustrated in Chapter 10, Fig. 10.9B). A thin membranous stenosis can often be lysed in the office using local anesthetic, but Gelfoam packing (Pfizer, Inc., New York, NY) in large strips should be placed for at least 2 weeks to prevent it from reforming. Residual cholesteatoma that forms behind a membranous partition will usually have to be removed in the operating room.

◆ Hearing Loss (Conductive and Neurosensory)

Conductive hearing loss is not uncommon after surgery, even in patients who have good hearing at the time of initial presentation. It is often the case that the cholesteatoma–ossicular complex transmits sound as a solid mass even with incus and stapes erosion. Conductive hearing loss should not be regarded as a true complication because removal of the incus or separation of the ossicular chain cannot be avoided in many cases, and the success of ossicular reconstruction is never certain. As discussed in Chapter 6, preservation of an intact ossicular chain should not take precedence over complete removal of disease. If the disease recurs, the eventual hearing outcome will almost surely decline.

Postoperative scarring with fibrosis of the middle ear, reduction of the size of the middle ear cleft because of lowering the posterior bony canal wall to the fallopian canal, and reducing the middle ear space can potentially prevent future middle ear hearing reconstruction.

Staging surgery is accepted when there is intact canal wall surgery in extensive cholesteatoma. Staging is also performed in patients with significant middle ear disease and eustachian tube dysfunction. At the first stage Silastic sheeting is frequently utilized to prevent middle ear fibrosis and help maintain a middle ear space. Second stage surgery may be performed under intravenous sedation, and the middle ear is entered, Silastic removed, and ossicular reconstruction performed. When it is necessary to remove the posterior canal wall, it is frequently possible to lower the canal wall just to the level of the chorda tympani inlet, still removing the sinus tympani or hypotympanum disease, therefore preserving a middle ear space for immediate or second-stage reconstruction. At a second stage the sheeting is removed and it is hoped that a middle ear cleft is retained. Then ossicular reconstruction may be performed under intravenous sedation technique.

A hearing aid can be offered to the patient once the ear is dry and stable. Bone-anchored hearing aid (BAHA, Cochlear Americas, Centennial, CO) is an option in chronically draining ears that cannot accept a hearing aid.[7] A BAHA provides excellent hearing results when the middle ear cannot be reconstructed and when bone conduction is good, but it requires a second operation to implant a titanium post and the use of an external processor. Round window implantation with the Vibrant device (MedEl, Durham, NC) is a newer option for hearing rehabilitation. This technique, in which a floating-mass transducer is placed against the round window membrane, introduced by Colletti et al[8] as a means of restoring hearing by bypassing the middle ear conductive mechanism, produced very encouraging initial hearing outcomes, although other authors have reported mixed results.[9]

Sensorineural hearing loss or deafness is fortunately not common after ear surgery. Preoperative sensorineural loss may be a feature of chronic middle ear infection, caused by the spread of inflammation to the inner ear. High-frequency postoperative sensorineural hearing loss occasionally occurs and may be undetected by the patient, but complete loss of hearing is a fairly serious complication. The incidence is increased when a fistula of the inner ear is present (labyrinthine or cochlear) from the disease, and especially in the presence of active infection. If a fistula is present at the time of surgery, the matrix should be kept on the fistula and canal wall down surgery performed, or rarely a second-stage surgery is performed with the matrix intact. At the second stage bony regrowth will occur. Iatrogenic opening of the inner ear

may occur if the semicircular canal is opened during drilling, or if the round window membrane is perforated during middle ear dissection, or if the annular ligament is broken while the surgeon is manipulating the stapes. When these events occur and are recognized during the surgery, immediate sealing of the inner ear with a fascial graft will usually prevent a significant cochlear loss.[10] The pathogenesis of sensorineural hearing loss in these cases may be toxic or suppurative labyrinthitis, perilymph leak, or inner ear fibrosis. When labyrinthitis occurs postoperatively, steroids may forestall the progression of sensorineural hearing loss, but once this has occurred it is probably irreversible.

High-frequency sensorineural hearing loss may result from vibrational trauma during drilling, particularly if the ossicular chain is intact. There is a potential for neurosensory hearing loss secondary to acoustic trauma of drilling (temporary or permanent threshold shift). Suction irrigation with drill sound may generate 100 dB levels for several minutes of drilling near the cochlea. There have been studies that have examined the pathophysiology of this phenomenon.[11,12] Vibrations transmitted through the skull bones are probably not sufficient to cause a permanent threshold shift, but drilling directly on the ossicular chain might be. To prevent this, care should be taken to avoid touching the drill to the ossicles in the attic (the cholesteatoma may provide a protective cushion), reducing the bone to an eggshell thickness that can be manually removed with a curette. Incus erosion is common in the presence of cholesteatoma, but sometimes an intact ossicular chain can be found even when the cholesteatoma is large. The status of the incudostapedial joint can be determined at the start of the case by raising a tympanomeatal flap, and it may be safer to separate the incudostapedial joint before drilling.[10]

◆ Tinnitus

Tinnitus in the early postoperative period may be related to middle ear swelling and often recovers when the surgical packing is removed. Patients who have tinnitus preoperatively may experience louder tinnitus postoperatively. Fortunately this is usually transient. High-pitched tinnitus is usually a manifestation of cochlear loss and may result from vibrational trauma. Tinnitus can be a vexing problem for patients and does not have an outright cure. Ambient masking is helpful, and a masking device may be beneficial for some patients. Benzodiazepines can alleviate anxiety and insomnia and often lessen the symptom. Tricyclic antidepressants (nortriptyline, amitriptyline) are also helpful and may act centrally to suppress tinnitus, rather than by an antidepressant effect.

◆ Dizziness and Imbalance

Dizziness and imbalance are not frequent. Like sensorineural loss, vestibular symptoms may arise from labyrinthitis or perilymph leakage. The chance of vertigo increases if an inner ear fistula is present. Vestibular symptoms may also result from surgical trauma to the inner ear, such as excessive manipulation of the stapes. Postoperative vertigo is usually transient and can be managed with vestibular suppressant medications such as meclizine, promethazine, or diazepam. Unilateral vestibular loss that is permanent generally recovers as central compensation takes hold. Imbalance will subside gradually and completely as activity is increased. Vestibular rehabilitation physical therapy may be helpful in cases that are slow to recover.

◆ Dysgeusia

Dysgeusia arises from surgical trauma to the chorda tympani nerve. Patients may complain of a metallic or altered taste on that side of the tongue, or dryness of the mouth. Its occurrence cannot be predicted. The chorda tympani is often enveloped by the cholesteatoma and must be sacrificed, and yet dysgeusia is not inevitable.[13] Stretch injury of the nerve may be more common than transection, and may result in greater symptoms.[14,15] Dysgeusia is usually temporary but may take 3 months or longer to resolve. In cases of bilateral chorda tympani sacrifice it may be permanent.

◆ Facial Paralysis

Facial paralysis is a dreaded complication that can arise from surgical trauma, the effect of local anesthesia, or the spread of infection to the nerve. It is more likely to occur when there is bony dehiscence of the fallopian canal, altered nerve anatomy, or extensive disease. The role of facial nerve monitoring and stimulation and the surgical technique of dissecting disease from the nerve have previously been covered. Proper technique demands an intimate knowledge of the course and anatomical position of the facial nerve. Monitoring is not a substitute for this.[16]

Most facial nerve injuries are first detected in the recovery room, not during the surgery.[17] If the paralysis is incomplete, then the nerve is probably not transected, and the function will probably recover. Note that complete (passive) eye closure may persist for > 24 hours after a facial nerve transection, and it is important not to be misled by this.[18] Partial or delayed facial nerve weakness should be treated with high-dose steroids, and both have a good prognosis for full recovery.

If a patient awakens from surgery with complete facial paralysis, the surgeon must consider where in the course of the operation an injury could have occurred (it is good surgical practice to identify the facial nerve in every otologic procedure).[19] If the disease was dissected off a bare nerve, the surgeon should have visualized the nerve and known the condition of the nerve at the end of the dissection. If the nerve was known to be intact and not mechanically traumatized, and if the nerve stimulator produced a good response with stimulus applied proximal to the site of the dissection, then it can be presumed that there was a neuropraxic injury with a very good chance of full spontaneous recovery. In most cases, however, the status of the nerve is not that certain, and urgent reexploration is advisable. In general, a transmastoid approach should be used (even if the original operation was

a tympanoplasty), and the entire nerve should be skeletonized from the first genu to the stylomastoid foramen.[20]

The area of nerve exposure should be inspected carefully. If the nerve appears intact but is edematous, a limited decompression of the bony canal should be conducted, using a small diamond drill, removing the bony covering both proximal and distal to the site of injury. The nerve stimulator should be applied proximal to the injury, starting at a low current level (0.05 mA) and increasing gradually to 2 mA until a response is obtained. Absence of response indicates severe neuropraxia and an uncertain prognosis. If the nerve is found to be disrupted, a limited decompression should similarly be undertaken, and the nerve stimulated proximally. If a response to stimulation is obtained, the nerve should be covered with a collagen sheath. If there is no response, the nerve should be carefully inspected. If less than 50% of the diameter of nerve is involved, the frayed edges should simply be reapproximated. If there is greater than 50% involvement, primary repair should be undertaken, either using fine sutures (9–0 nylon or Prolene, Ethicon, Inc., Somerville, NJ) through the epineurial sheath or coapting the ends in the bony fallopian canal. If a section of the nerve is missing, an interposition graft should be taken from the great auricular nerve. The time course of return of function will be days to weeks for a neuropraxic injury, 6 to 12 months for a severed nerve in the middle ear. Neuropraxia will generally recover fully, whereas a nerve repair will usually result in partial recovery (House-Brackmann grade 3). It is very important to counsel the patient and family of the expected outcome, and to remain involved in the patient's care during the postoperative period.[21] Eye protection is important to prevent corneal dryness, and a lid-loading gold weight procedure[22] may be beneficial if a long period of recovery is likely.

◆ Vascular Injury

The sigmoid sinus, internal jugular vein, and internal carotid artery are susceptible to surgical injury. The neurotologic skull base surgeon usually possesses firsthand experience in approaching and handling these structures, but the general otolaryngologist who operates on the ear may not. It is important therefore to know what to do if a vascular injury does arise.

The sigmoid sinus is usually identified anatomically during mastoidectomy. There is a thin plate of bone overlying the sinus, and in cholesteatoma surgery this should be maintained. A cutting burr can be used to skeletonize the sigmoid provided the surgeon keeps a very light hand, but a diamond burr is safer. The sinus is a dural structure, and removing the bony covering does not necessarily lead to venous injury, but this may happen if the sinus is thin or bulging.

Lacerating the sigmoid sinus causes profuse venous bleeding, of course, and the surgeon should be equipped to deal with this. The first measure is to control the bleeding with external pressure, using oxidized cellulose (Surgicel, Ethicon, Inc., Somerville NJ) gauze, a neurosurgical cottonoid, or even finger pressure. The bleeding can then be definitively controlled using an extraluminal plug of Gelfoam (Pfizer, Inc., New York, NY) soaked in thrombin. Using a 5F Baron suction in the nondominant hand to divert the blood, the Surgicel is slowly peeled away until the bleeding site is visualized. If it is very small it can be controlled with bipolar cautery. If it is 1 or 2 mm in size, a Gelfoam-thrombin plug can be gently inserted into the opening. If it is larger than 2 mm, a square of Gelfoam-thrombin can be placed extraluminally and held in place by sandwiching it between the edges of the bony opening and the sinus wall.[23] This requires gently separating the dura from the bone with a blunt duckbill elevator prior to placing the packing. A still larger tear, should it ever occur, might require obliterating the sinus with extraluminal Surgicel packing, but this situation should be avoided if at all possible. Intraluminal packing should be avoided because it can embolize toward the heart; if this is ever necessary, the internal jugular vein should be ligated in the neck.[20]

The jugular bulb can also bleed if treated roughly, and bleeding from the jugular is handled in the same way. The jugular is encountered in two places—in the hypotympanum through the middle ear, and in the retrofacial cell tract through the mastoid. The jugular bulb is highly variable in position. A high jugular bulb can be injured during seemingly innocuous maneuvers, such as elevating a tympanomeatal flap, if it lies in a vulnerable location.

The internal carotid artery is not often encountered during surgery for chronic ear disease, and injury to the carotid is rare. The carotid can be reliably found medial to the eustachian tube in the protympanum. The bony wall there is thin or can be absent, placing the carotid at risk in that location. The carotid has a thick muscular wall. Surgical injury when it occurs results from penetrating trauma; sharp instrumentation should therefore be avoided in that area. A laceration of the carotid artery will cause dramatic pulsatile bleeding. Temporary control can be gained with extraluminal pressure; definitive control will require an endovascular procedure performed by an interventional neuroradiologist. In a dire emergency, ligation of the internal carotid artery in the neck might be required.

◆ Cerebrospinal Fluid Leak

Cerebrospinal fluid (CSF) leakage is an uncommon but potentially serious complication because it can lead to meningitis. CSF leakage can result from removal of cholesteatoma matrix from thin dura or from surgical trauma during drilling. The tegmen is the most vulnerable site. Spontaneous dural dehiscences occur in at least 20% of chronic ears, and small encephaloceles are even more vulnerable to surgical trauma. CSF leakage can also occur spontaneously in association with arachnoid granulations, intracranial hypertension, meningoencephaloceles, or congenital inner ear anomalies. Once a CSF leak is discovered, it is imperative to repair it. Small dural tears can usually be repaired through a transmastoid approach, as described in Chapter 6. A multilayer repair using fascia and conchal cartilage in the epidural space will usually be successful. Occasionally it may be necessary to use one of the manufactured onlay synthetic dural repair substances, which are conformable and resorbable membrane with collagen. (ie, Durepair, Medtronic Sofamor Danek, Inc., Memphis, TN; DuraMatrix Stryker,

Kalamazoo, MI; DuraGen, Integra NeuroScience, Plainsboro, NJ) Rarely, the mastoid cavity may have to be packed with abdominal fat in a canal wall up procedure. It is very important when obliterating the mastoid to be certain that no residual disease remains. In a canal wall down, the area of leakage will be open to the outside. The option exists of obliterating the ear with fat and oversewing the meatus, but this will compromise hearing as well as postoperative surveillance. Hydroxyapatite bone cement can also be used but must be completely covered with a soft tissue flap prior to closure. Large encephaloceles, multiple dural tears, or leaks that are inaccessible from below can be repaired via transcranial route. This can be done through an extradural approach using a middle fossa craniotomy (or minicraniotomy), elevating the dura bluntly until the area of the dural tear is reached. An oversized fascia graft can then be sandwiched into the epidural space, and a piece of cartilage, split calvarial bone, or hydroxyapatite disc can be used to repair the tegmen from above. These measures will control most CSF leaks. In cases of profuse or recurrent leaks, a lumbar drain can be inserted for 3 to 5 days to reduce CSF pressure and allow the defect to seal, and an intradural repair can be performed via temporal craniotomy by the neurosurgeon, although not usually necessary.

◆ Conclusion

Cholesteatoma surgery is challenging, and even the most experienced surgeon may encounter complications. The neurosensory organs and vascular structures of the temporal bone require delicate and precise surgical technique. Preparedness in knowing how to deal with problems in the operating room and in the postoperative period is essential to maximizing surgical outcomes.

References

1. Kos MI, Castrillon R, Montandon P, Guyot JP. Anatomic and functional long-term results of canal wall-down mastoidectomy. Ann Otol Rhinol Laryngol 2004;113(11):872–876
2. Jackson CG, Schall DG, Glasscock ME III, Macias JD, Widick MH, Touma BJ. A surgical solution for the difficult chronic ear. Am J Otol 1996;17(1): 7–14
3. Ramsey MJ, Merchant SN, McKenna MJ. Postauricular periosteal-pericranial flap for mastoid obliteration and canal wall down tympano-mastoidectomy. Otol Neurotol 2004;25(6):873–878
4. Paparella MM, Meyerhoff WL. "How I do it"—otology and neurology: a specific issue and its solution. Meatoplasty. Laryngoscope 1978;88(2 Pt 1):357–359
5. Sheehy JL, Glasscock ME III. Tympanic membrane grafting with temporalis fascia. Arch Otolaryngol 1967;86(4):391–402
6. Hough JV. Revision tympanoplasty including anterior perforations and lateralization of grafts. Otolaryngol Clin North Am 2006;39(4): 661–675, v
7. Macnamara M, Phillips D, Proops DW. The bone anchored hearing aid (BAHA) in chronic suppurative otitis media (CSOM). J Laryngol Otol Suppl 1996;21:38–40
8. Colletti V, Carner M, Colletti L. TORP vs round window implant for hearing restoration of patients with extensive ossicular chain defect. Acta Otolaryngol 2009;129(4):449–452
9. Beltrame AM, Martini A, Prosser S, Giarbini N, Streitberger C. Coupling the Vibrant Soundbridge to cochlea round window: auditory results in patients with mixed hearing loss. Otol Neurotol 2009;30(2):194–201

10. Palva T, Kärjä J, Palva A. Immediate and short-term complications of chronic ear surgery. Arch Otolaryngol 1976;102(3):137–139

11. Urquhart AC, McIntosh WA, Bodenstein NP. Drill-generated sensorineural hearing loss following mastoid surgery. Laryngoscope 1992;102(6):689–692

12. Migirov L, Wolf M. Influence of drilling on the distortion product otoacoustic emissions in the non-operated ear. ORL J Otorhinolaryngol Relat Spec 2009;71(3):153–156

13. Clark MPA, O'Malley S. Chorda tympani nerve function after middle ear surgery. Otol Neurotol 2007;28(3):335–340

14. Gopalan P, Kumar M, Gupta D, Phillipps JJ. A study of chorda tympani nerve injury and related symptoms following middle-ear surgery. J Laryngol Otol 2005;119(3):189–192

15. Michael P, Raut V. Chorda tympani injury: operative findings and postoperative symptoms. Otolaryngol Head Neck Surg 2007;136(6):978–981

16. Prass RL. Iatrogenic facial nerve injury: the role of facial nerve monitoring. Otolaryngol Clin North Am 1996;29(2):265–275

17. Green JD Jr, Shelton C, Brackmann DE. Surgical management of iatrogenic facial nerve injuries. Otolaryngol Head Neck Surg 1994;111(5):606–610

18. Graham MD. Prevention and management of iatrogenic facial palsy. Am J Otol 1984;5(6):513

19. Glasscock ME III, Wiet RJ, Jackson CG, Dickins JR. Rehabilitation of the face following traumatic injury to the facial nerve. Laryngoscope 1979;89(9 Pt 1):1389–1404

20. Weber PC. Iatrogenic complications from chronic ear surgery. Otolaryngol Clin North Am 2005;38(4):711–722

21. Pulec JL. Iatrogenic facial palsy: the cost. Ear Nose Throat J 1996;75(11):730–736

22. Bojrab DI. ___ Insights in Otolaryngology 1989;4(4):1–5

23. Brackmann DE. Iatrogenic injuries in temporal bone surgery. In: Britton BH, ed. Common Problems in Otology. St. Louis: Mosby; 1991:115–119

Index

Note: Page numbers followed by *f* and *t* indicate figures and tables, respectively.